"I Flunked My PSA!"

What you need to know about prostate cancer

NOW!

"I Flunked My PSA!"

What you need to know about prostate cancer

NOW!

Ernie Bodai, M.D., F.A.C.S.
Surgeon and Prostate Cancer Survivor

with
Richard A. Zmuda

B2Z Publishing, Inc.
Severna Park, Maryland

Copyright © 2002 Ernie Bodai, MD and Richard A. Zmuda

All rights reserved. No part of this book shall be reproduced, stored in a retrieval system or transmitted by any means, electronic, mechanical, photocopying, recording or otherwise, without written permission from the publisher.

"I Flunked My PSA!" is a registered trademark of B2Z Publishing.

International Standard Book Number (ISBN): 0-9712070-1-1
Library of Congress Catalog Card Number: Available upon request.

Printed in the United States of America.

Note: The information contained herein is for educational purposes only and is intended to provide helpful information to men facing a significant prostate cancer risk or who are undergoing treatment for the disease. The authors have used extensive efforts to ensure that the information is accurate and current. However, advances in medical research and treatment may invalidate certain information. Any person who has or might have a health problem should consult a professional healthcare provider.

B2Z Publishing, Inc.
Post Office Box 307
Severna Park, Maryland 21146 USA
Tel: 1-888-371-1800 (toll free) / 410-431-8894
Web site: www.B2Zpublishing.com
E-mail: towardcure@aol.com

A portion of the proceeds from each book will be donated by the authors to support prostate cancer education programs.

The cover depicts a broken DNA strand and the revolutionary efforts by individual researchers to repair it. Also shown, courtesy of the U.S. Postal Service, is the Prostate Cancer Awareness Stamp, which was issued in 1999.

Cover design and illustration on page 6 by Joshua D. Williams.

Illustrations on page 35 and in Appendix I courtesy of Aventis Oncology.

Dedication

To the cancer angels who
watch over us all ...

You know who you are.

Foreword

By Michael Milken

Philanthropist, Financier, Prostate Cancer Survivor
Founder of CaP CURE—The Association for the Cure
of Cancer of the Prostate

This book contains hundreds of useful facts that will help you understand prostate cancer. But there's one overriding fact you should keep in mind—a diagnosis of prostate cancer is never a reason to lose hope. Treatments are improving all the time. Millions of prostate cancer survivors are living full, satisfying and productive lives.

I was diagnosed in 1993 and had already spent the better part of two decades learning about cancer and supporting a broad range of medical research through my family's foundation. Sadly, many members of my family had succumbed to various forms of cancer, including breast cancer and malignant melanoma. In thinking about what I could do that my relatives had not done, it became clear that they hadn't really taken charge of their cases, probably because they lacked sufficient information. And although it seemed that I had spent a lifetime dealing with cancer, I didn't have much information about prostate cancer. So I started studying the disease and soon learned about the challenges ahead.

In the United States, about 43,000 men died from prostate cancer in 1993. The death toll was expected to rise to 55,000 partly because of the continued increase in aging baby boomers. Newspapers and magazines carried relatively few articles about the disease. Young physicians and scientists were advised not to pursue careers in prostate cancer research because little money was available for their investigations. Doctors at comprehensive cancer centers rarely communicated their findings to each other. There were almost no clinical trials of new drugs and treatments. Researchers were often unable to obtain samples of tumors for testing new compounds. Nutrition as a field of serious research was largely ignored. Finally, like breast cancer a generation earlier, prostate cancer was still "in the closet," something that wasn't discussed in polite society.

Once the shock of my own diagnosis had subsided, I determined to do something about the situation. That was the beginning of CaP CURE, which started with a threefold mission: to support medical research that will translate into treatments and cures for a broad range of serious diseases; to advance understanding of all forms of human cancer; and to identify and support prostate cancer research with the potential to vanquish this devastating disease. We quickly hired a talented professional staff and began to figure out how to accelerate research, which was often bogged down in bureaucracy and red tape. We simplified and speeded up the grant process and gave the first of what are now nearly 1,000 research grants that have led to more than 80 human clinical trials of promising new treatments.

In 1994, CaP CURE hosted the first of its annual Scientific Retreats, now an important professional forum for researchers and clinicians from around the world. We've also been active in Washington by encouraging the exchange of information about cancer among all government branches. In 1995, we organized the first National Cancer Summit. Later, Congress passed legislation that speeds up approval of new drugs. In 1998, "The March: Coming Together to Conquer Cancer" drew hundreds of thousands of marchers to Washington and other cities to demonstrate for more research funding.

By 2001, government outlays for prostate cancer research reached $550 million, up from only $27 million in 1993. It is important to note, however, that medical research is not a zero-sum game where support for one disease area diminishes support of others. We should be working to conquer all serious diseases by funding basic research in addition to expanding the entire pie for applied research.

Today, young scientists and physicians entering the field of prostate cancer research have much broader options than just a decade ago. CaP CURE leads a Therapy Consortium in which research leaders exchange information several times a year. We've also established a nationwide tissue bank and helped identify families that carry useful cell lines. Our research has validated the worth of nutritional approaches by indicating strong associations between diet and cancer. More men are getting tested earlier and nearly 20,000 articles about prostate cancer are being published every year—an eight-fold increase over 1993. Our web site, www.capcure.org, has become a valued resource for patients and for doctors and other professionals seeking the latest information on research progress.

But most importantly, all of this has contributed to a reduced death rate, down 28% to 31,500 in nine years. While we can't relax our efforts until the death rate drops to zero, you should know that the odds are improving every day. You can improve your own odds by using the information in this book to help you take charge of your treatments. Information is empowering and with Dr. Bodai's book, you have the power to work with your own doctor toward a successful outcome.

Michael Milken

Acknowledgments

"I Flunked My PSA!" would not have been possible without the extraordinary support of so many wonderful individuals. We feel privileged to have been able to work with the following medical specialists who are, in our opinion, without peer:

Larry Goldman, M.D.
Director, Sacramento Brachytherapy
Kaiser Permanente, Sacramento

Manouchehr Lalehzarian, M.D., F.A.C.S.
Chairman, Prostate Cancer Awareness and Education in California
Department of Urology, Kaiser Permanente, Fontana

Daryl Lance, Pharma.D.
Oncologic Pharmacologist
Kaiser Permanente, Sacramento

Primo N. Lara, Jr., M.D.
Assistant Professor of Medicine
University of California Davis Cancer Center, Sacramento

David Lindstadt, M.D.
Chief, Radiation Oncology
Sutter Roseville Medical Center
Assistant Clinical Professor of Radiation Oncology
University of California, San Francisco

In addition, we gratefully acknowledge the *invaluable* contributions of: **Stan Rosenfeld**, a prostate cancer survivor who provided important insight from a patient's perspective; **Phyllis Avedon**, for her extraordinary editorial skills; and **Jean Chew, Therese Nakata, Erlinda Patterson, Jami Turner** and **Helene Wolf** for their patience and support throughout all phases of this endeavor.

About the Author

The wealth of medical information available to men with prostate cancer is often far too complex and sometimes even misleading for the average patient, according to Dr. Ernie Bodai, a nationally renowned breast cancer surgeon who is also a prostate cancer survivor.

There has long been a need for an easy-to-read yet thorough "prostate cancer primer" that could explain the disease in a way that the vast majority of prostate cancer patients can understand. To address this issue, he wrote *"I Flunked My PSA!" What you need to know about prostate cancer NOW!*

Since his prostate cancer diagnosis in 2000, Dr. Bodai has become a passionate advocate for prostate cancer in the same way that, as a breast cancer surgeon, he championed the hugely successful U.S. Postal Service (USPS) Breast Cancer Research Stamp, which has already raised more than $30 million toward crucial research into that disease.

Dr. Bodai is currently working with the USPS to produce a similar stamp for prostate cancer, but a decision will not be made for several years. In the interim, he continues to testify non-stop at both the state and national levels for increased funding for prostate cancer research.

Prostate and breast cancer are, in many ways, mirror-image diseases. The statistics for both, as well as diagnosis, treatment, survival and issues of intimacy, are remarkably similar. Dr. Bodai now has *two* missions: attempting to irradicate *both* prostate and breast cancer.

Given his track record, we believe he will succeed.

Preface

Healing Takes Time

It all began with a concern, a symptom, or your PSA was suspicious. That's the first time the word "cancer" entered your mind. Sure, it happens to some people. But to me?

You start getting anxious; you want answers immediately. But answers often take time. So do follow-up tests, or the results of a biopsy. Initially you weren't concerned, but you are beginning to wonder if everything will be all right.

Then you find out you have prostate cancer! What was originally nothing more than a routine annual check-up has turned into a long and uncertain journey. Things on your "To Do" list that seemed immensely important only a few days ago have suddenly become irrelevant. New tests are ordered; you now have to wait for *these* results.

At the same time, you have to gather up all of your courage to tell your loved ones—not only that you have prostate cancer, but that everything will be okay. (You wonder, will it?) Everyone will want to know what is happening to you, but you don't even know yourself!

STOP!

Take a deep breath. You have time to gather your thoughts, to make informed decisions.

You don't have to become an immediate expert on everything remotely related to prostate cancer. It is important, however, to have a general understanding of the disease that is now confronting you, and to fully comprehend the treatment options that are available. This book will help, as will innumerable discussions with your healthcare team in the coming months.

There will be lots of "waiting" throughout your treatment regimen: waiting for the next doctor's appointment; waiting for a return phone call; waiting for lab results. Treatment will eventually start—you can't wait till it ends. You can't wait to feel better!

With each wait, your anxiety and stress levels increase. You sense a "loss of control," that the treatment is taking over your life.

But it doesn't have to. In fact, *you* are in control—every step of the way. Yes, you have to confront this disease, but you can do so on your own terms.

First, accept the fact that the treatment and recovery process takes time. Answers will come, treatments will succeed. Never as quickly as you would like, but they will.

Second, establish good relationships with your healthcare team—your surgeon, oncologist, radiologist, nurses, social workers and others. Always communicate *any* concerns that you have. Remember that all treatment decisions are *your* decisions.

Finally, establish a support system. This could involve other men who have been through a similar experience, family members, close friends, clergy or social workers. You will soon find that others want to help, *need* to help. Allow them to. You do not have to go through this alone.

It is easy to say, "Just relax and don't worry." But you won't relax—and of course you will worry. Nonetheless, you *will* get through this. It won't be easy at times. But you will. And in some very important ways, you will come out the better for it. You will forever appreciate the simple joys that life affords, and the special people who have always been there for you.

Most importantly, you may discover an extraordinary inner strength that you did not realize you had. As the poet E.E. Cummings once wrote:

> "In the midst of winter I suddenly learned
> that there was within me an invincible summer!"

Heal well. Stay well!

Ernie Bodai and Richard Zmuda

"I Flunked My PSA!"

What you need to know about prostate cancer NOW!

INTRODUCTION

A Prostate Cancer Primer 5
No Single Cause 8

PART I: RISK FACTORS AND SCREENING

Risk Factors 13
Age 14
Race 15
Genetic Risk 15
Diet 16
Hormones 17
Additional Factors 17

Prevention? 21
Exercise 21
Diet 22
Finasteride: The Prostate Cancer Prevention Trial 23
Selenium and Vitamin E: The SELECT Trial 24
Preventing Cancer with Vitamins and Minerals 25
Cancer Vaccines 27
Risk Reduction 28

Screening Techniques 31
Digital Rectal Exam 31
Prostate-Specific Antigen (PSA) 32
Other Screening Tests 32
    - Transrectal Ultrasonography 33
    - Prostatic Acid Phosphatase 33
    - Biopsy 33
False Positive/False Negative Results 33
New Screening Techniques 34
    - Free PSA 34
    - PSA Velocity 34
    - Age-Adjusted PSA 34
    - PSA Density 34
Minority Screening 36
Benign (Non-Cancerous) Prostate Conditions 38
The Prostate, Lung, Colorectal, and Ovarian Screening Trial 39

PART II: DIAGNOSIS AND TREATMENT

A Diagnosis of Cancer: What Does It Mean? 43
Recognizing Symptoms 44
Stages of Prostate Cancer 45
The Gleason Score 46
Family and Friends are Impacted Too 46
Speak Up During Doctor Visits 48
Talking To Your Kids 49
Second Opinions 50

Understanding Your Treatment Options 53
Watchful Waiting 53
    - Side Effects of Watchful Waiting 54
Surgery 55
    - Side Effects of Surgery 56
Radiation Therapy 57
    - Side Effects of Radiation Therapy 59
Hormonal Therapy 61
    - Side Effects of Hormonal Therapy 62

Treatment Options: Choosing Between Them 63
New Treatments on the Horizon 63
The Prostate Cancer Outcomes Study 64
Complementary and Alternative Therapies 65
Clinical Trials 69
A Few Words About Pain 71
Treatment Follow-Up 72

PART III: RECOVERY

Emotional Issues 78
Intimacy and Sexuality 78
Financial Issues 79
Cancer and Your Career 80
Changing Jobs 81
Personal Support 82
Support Groups 83
Coping with Recurrence 84
Living with Advanced Disease 84

APPENDICES

Appendix I: Stages of Prostate Cancer 89
Appendix II: Prostate Cancer Treatment Options 97
Appendix III: Common Prostate Cancer Drugs
 – Hormonal Agents 107
Appendix IV: Common Prostate Cancer Drugs
 – Chemotherapy Agents 111
Appendix V: Common Anti-Nausea Medications 115
Appendix VI: Prostate Cancer and Sexuality 119
Appendix VII: Glossary of Prostate Cancer Terms. 131
Appendix VIII: Off the Bookshelf 143
Appendix IX: Internet Resources 151
Appendix X: National Organizations 157

INDEX 163

Introduction

Most men aren't aware of a startling statistic – "One out of six men will get prostate cancer in their lifetime." Unfortunately, *you* are now that one out of six. You certainly didn't choose to be, but you are.

As such, here is the statistic that you should *now* focus on: **Close to 95 percent of men whose prostate cancer is caught in its earliest stages will be healthy and disease-free five years after their diagnosis and treatment.** Even if your prostate cancer was not caught early, the outlook is extremely promising. In fact, **the five-year survival rate for ALL men with prostate cancer still exceeds 85 percent!**

Major advances in prostate cancer screening techniques are just around the corner, which will enable us to detect prostate tumors at much smaller sizes. New anti-cancer drugs are emerging from clinical trials, and the revolutionary decoding of the human DNA sequence will eventually lead to the elimination of cancer as a life-threatening illness. Cancer may still occur, but it will no longer be the medical challenge that it is today.

You already have at your disposal an extraordinary array of treatments, many of which did not exist a decade ago. Your cancer *can* be beaten. It's not just hype. It's hope, and it's here.

A Prostate Cancer Primer

The prostate is a gland in a man's reproductive system. It makes and stores *seminal fluid*, a milky substance that nourishes sperm. This fluid is released to form a major component of *semen*. The prostate is about the size of a walnut. It is located below the *bladder* and in front of the *rectum*. It surrounds the upper part of the *urethra*, which is the

"I Flunked My PSA!"

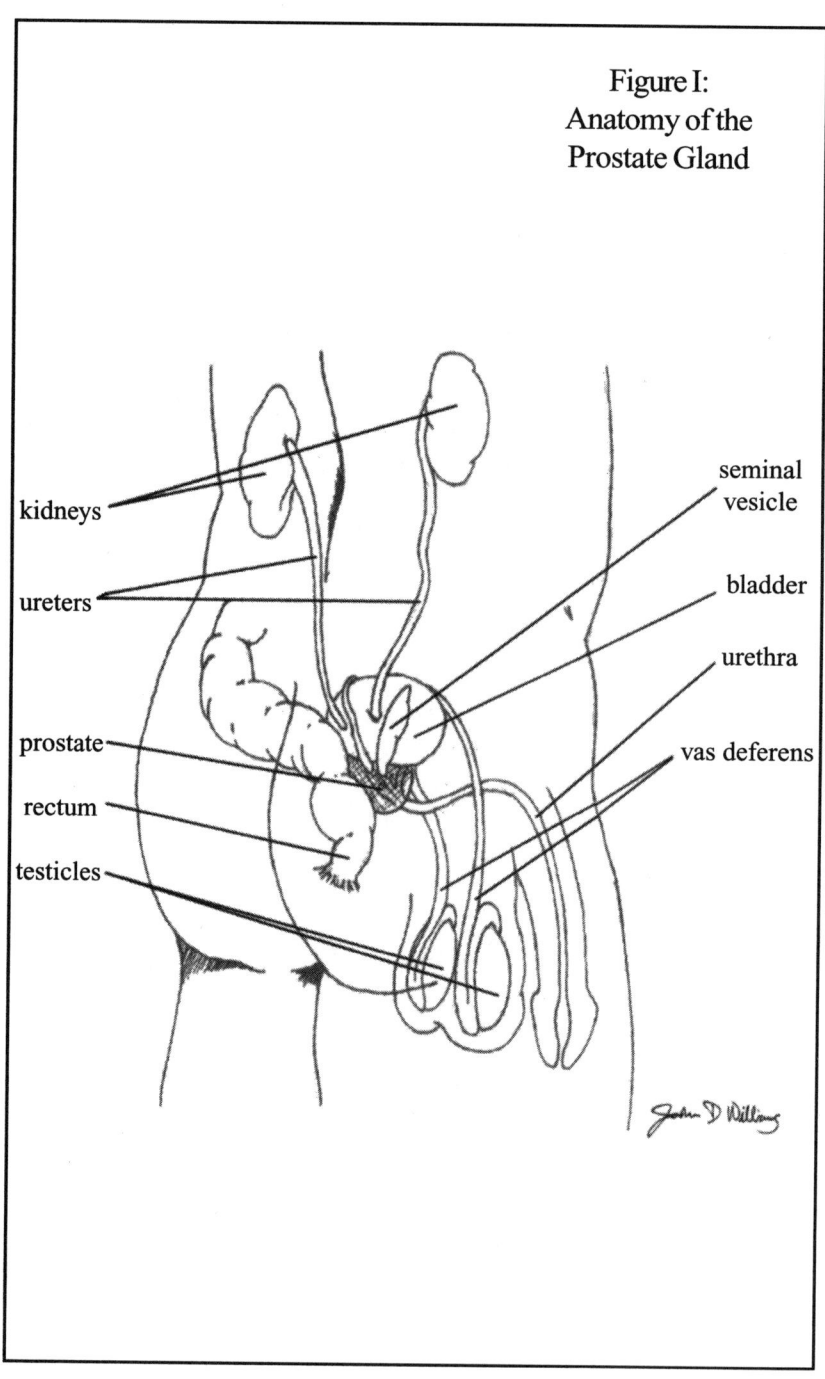

Figure I: Anatomy of the Prostate Gland

tube that empties urine from the bladder. (See Figure I.)

The prostate enlarges as you get older. However, if the prostate grows too large, the flow of urine can be slowed or even stopped altogether. This is a common complaint for men after age 50 and is not considered a sign of prostate cancer.

To work properly, the prostate needs male *hormones* (*androgens*). Male hormones are responsible for male sexual characteristics. The main male hormone or androgen is *testosterone*, which is made mostly by the *testicles*. Some male hormones are produced in smaller amounts by the *adrenal glands*, which are located above each kidney.

Except for skin cancer, cancer of the prostate is the most common cancer in American men. It is estimated that in 2002 in the United States nearly 200,000 men will be diagnosed with prostate cancer. Fortunately, prostate cancer is a relatively slow-growing cancer. In fact, because of this slow growth rate, "watchful waiting" (close follow-up to see if the cancer grows) is a legitimate treatment alternative for some patients.

What exactly is cancer?

The actual word "cancer" is confusing. It is a catch-all term for diseases that are characterized by the uncontrolled growth of cells. The exact type of cancer that a person has is categorized by its origin; in your case it is *prostate* cancer because it originated in the prostate gland. Even if the cancer spreads (*metastasizes*) from the prostate to the bones or lymph nodes, it is still referred to as "prostate cancer," not bone cancer or lymphatic cancer.

Basically, a cancer cell is a cell that just doesn't know when or how to stop growing or dividing. All cells have a natural lifespan, but sometimes a cell won't die when its time is up. The cell may have been altered by some outside factor or, in the case of inherited cancers, a mutation in its genetic code may have been passed down from earlier generations, causing it to keep dividing and growing.

The cancer cell divides into two cancer cells, then four, then eight, and so on. Eventually, there are hundreds and then thousands of them clustering together to form a lump or mass (called a tumor).

Cancer doesn't just appear overnight; it takes years to develop to a detectable stage. Once it grows to a certain level, it expands exponentially. If left unchecked, these out-of-control cells eventually spread to nearby tissues, and then to other tissues and organs farther away. While this process usually takes a long time, we are nonetheless in a hurry to treat the disease.

Cancerous cells can spread to other parts of the body in a number of ways: they can grow into a mass (tumor) and invade nearby tissues or organs; or they can break away and spread through the bloodstream or the *lymphatic* system to other parts of the body. The lymphatic system is composed of many channels dispersed throughout the body; it is responsible for cleansing the blood. Lymph nodes are tiny "filters" located within the channels that remove toxins and foreign substances from surrounding tissues.

A tumor is an abnormal collection of cells. A prostate tumor can be a *benign* (non-cancerous) enlargement that occurs with aging, or *malignant* (cancerous). A benign tumor can be treated and in most cases will not come back. A malignant tumor can grow and affect nearby tissues or can break away and travel to distant parts of the body.

No Single Cause

Only 5 to 10 percent of prostate cancers are hereditary; that is, they are caused by a faulty gene that has been passed down from generation to generation. The majority of prostate cancers are caused by something else. Many theories have been proposed, all of which have their supporters. But today we still do not know exactly what causes prostate cancer.

Age is clearly a predominant risk factor for prostate cancer.

Introduction

More than three-quarters of men diagnosed with the disease each year are over the age of 65. Because of increased public awareness and improved screening, the age at diagnosis continues to decrease.

In addition, race appears to play a role—African-American men have a 60 percent greater risk of developing prostate cancer than Caucasian men. The disparity is even more pronounced when compared with men of Asian descent.

Some researchers believe that a high-fat diet may also play a role in the development of prostate cancer. Others have focused on a lack of exercise, smoking, exposure to certain sexually transmitted viruses—the list goes on and on. In fact, prostate cancer is likely the result of a combination of factors.

* * * * * * * * *

Having said all of this, here you are—either facing a significant risk of prostate cancer, or possibly having just been diagnosed. You may even be on the welcome road to recovery.

Whatever the reason, you now have this book in your hands and have therefore taken an important first step. We are going to help you take many more.

PART I:

Risk Factors and Screening

Risk Factors

"I already HAVE prostate cancer," you might say. "So why should I worry about risk factors NOW?"

On the surface, it does seem odd. However, unless you have a strong family history of prostate cancer, you may never know exactly what caused your cancer. Therefore, as you move beyond treatment and recovery toward a long and healthy life, you will clearly want to do everything you can to minimize the risk of the cancer coming back (*recurring*).

A recent survey of European women with breast cancer found that only nine percent of them believed that an unhealthy diet contributed to their disease. Yet nearly a third of the women significantly changed their dietary habits after their diagnosis. Why? The better question is, why not?

Many of the women reduced their consumption of fat, sugar and red meat; they began eating more fruits and vegetables and started taking vitamin supplements. This was especially true for younger women. The researchers suggested that these dietary changes represented a way for the women to exert some form of influence over their own well-being.

They were right! Keep in mind that you *always* have some influence over factors affecting not only your cancer risk, but also your overall health. As these women would tell you, it simply can't hurt to improve your diet, exercise more, and generally take better care of yourself. While this study addressed women with breast cancer, the same principles apply to men with prostate cancer as well.

Such changes will have benefits far beyond reducing your risk factors for cancer. You'll feel stronger, healthier, have a more positive outlook on life, and possibly avoid dozens of *other* ailments that directly result from an unhealthy lifestyle.

What about a family history of prostate cancer, something that is totally out of your control? Does that put you at greater risk? Yes, it definitely does. But what if you have *no* family history of prostate cancer. Does that mean that you are off the hook? Unfortunately, no.

The vast majority of newly diagnosed prostate cancer patients have no known history of the disease in their family. Keep in mind that the last generation often did not discuss sensitive issues such as prostate cancer, and important diagnostic tests were not available 20 or 30 years ago. Many of us, therefore, may have had a close relative with prostate cancer, but simply have no knowledge of it.

Age

Probably the single most important risk factor for prostate cancer is age. Prostate cancer is found mainly in men over the age of 55. In fact, about 97 percent of prostate cancer cases are diagnosed in men 55 and older. More than three quarters of all newly diagnosed prostate cancer cases occur in men age 65 and older.

Because it is detected almost exclusively at an older age, prostate cancer is unique amongst cancers, most of which may occur earlier in life. There is great debate between researchers about whether this age factor results because prostate cancer is a very slow-growing cancer (which makes "watchful waiting" a viable treatment strategy), or whether something involved in the natural aging process may act as its trigger.

Whatever the link between age and prostate cancer, it is extremely important for men, particularly those over the age of 50, to have regular screening, which includes an annual digital rectal exam and PSA (Prostate–Specific Antigen) blood test. Men with a family history of prostate cancer and African-American men should actually begin screening ten years earlier. All men should establish a baseline

PSA level at an early age so that any changes or trends can be readily acted upon.

Race

Prostate cancer is much more common in African-American men than in any other racial or ethnic group. The incidence is roughly 60 percent higher among African Americans than Caucasians; this gap is even wider when compared with Asian Americans.

There may be some unknown biological differences in the way prostate cancer tumors develop in African-American men. Research is focusing on certain proteins that are more abundant in these tumors. No conclusive findings are available, in part hampered by the disproportionately low participation of African Americans and other minorities in clinical trials.

It may be years until we can pinpoint why this glaring racial disparity exists—and be able to develop new risk reduction methods and treatments to counteract it. Until then, it is essential that African-American men be especially vigilant about regular screening. While screening techniques are readily available, getting the message out to African-American men continues to be a challenge.

Genetic Risk

Genes are the basic units of heredity—affecting characteristics that are passed down from generation to generation. They determine obvious traits, such as facial features, eye and hair color, as well as more subtle ones, such as the oxygen-carrying ability of blood. It is estimated that humans have approximately 100,000 genes, but a flaw in *any one* of them could result in some specific disease.

Studies have shown that only 5 to 10 percent of all prostate cancers are caused by hereditary factors such as a strong family history of the disease. The vast majority of prostate cancers, therefore, cannot be linked to a genetic origin.

However, if you have family members who have had prostate cancer, especially if they developed the disease at a younger age, you are definitely at higher risk. Some studies have suggested that as many as 40 percent of prostate cancers in men younger than age 55 may have a genetic basis.

New research is now focusing on a possible link between prostate cancer and mutations in the so-called breast cancer genes—BRCA1 (BReast CAncer I) and BRCA2. Some researchers believe you are at an increased risk if you have relatives with either prostate cancer *or* breast cancer. Further studies are needed to clarify this relationship.

If you have a family history of prostate (or possibly breast) cancer, you need to disclose this to your doctor. He or she may suggest seeing a healthcare professional trained in genetics.

Diet

There are Asian diets rich in soy, olive oil-laden Mediterranean diets, low-fat diets, vegetarian diets. The headlines are full of stories touting the newest cancer-fighting cuisines; such recommendations seem to change on a weekly basis.

In all likelihood, diet may play a role in the onset of some cancers, including prostate cancer. Results from several major studies have shown that the rates of prostate cancer in certain countries are far lower than those in the United States. Is a healthier diet the reason? Or is it the consumption of certain culture-specific foods? Studies to date have not been conclusive, yet the data appear to be far too convincing to ignore.

For example, the incidence of prostate cancer has been rising in Japan, where substantial dietary changes have occurred in the past three decades. Diets have become more "Westernized," especially with higher fat intake. Also, the incidence of prostate cancer rises in Japanese and Chinese immigrants the longer they reside in the United States.

The main dietary component that has been associated with prostate cancer is fat. Unfortunately, obesity is at an all-time high in the United States. This unhealthy situation may be responsible for *many* health-related problems, including a higher rate of prostate cancer. According to the American Obesity Association, 22 percent of the total adult U.S. population—39 million people—meet the criteria for obesity.

Whether you have cancer or not, a healthier diet that is low in fat and high in fruits and vegetables is a great first step toward minimizing the risk of prostate cancer or its recurrence. And why not throw in a little soy or olive oil in the process? It certainly can't hurt, and it may taste good too!

Hormones

Some research suggests that high levels of the male hormone androgen may increase the risk of prostate cancer. Androgens are required for the normal growth and development of healthy prostate cells, but these same hormones may in turn fuel the growth of prostate *cancer* cells. Unfortunately, current research has been inconclusive.

New studies are trying to identify the specific genes that control various aspects of androgen production and whether some of these are involved in the disparate rates of prostate cancer among African-American men.

Additional Factors

The headlines are constantly touting the cancer-fighting properties of this fruit or that vegetable, or telling us of a new "prostate cancer risk factor" that has just been identified. Be wary.

A few studies have suggested that having a *vasectomy* might increase a man's risk for developing prostate cancer, but more current research does not support this finding. Other studies are evaluating whether a non-cancerous condition called benign prostatic hyperplasia (BPH)—enlargement of the prostate—may be a precursor to prostate cancer; still others are focusing on a lack of exercise, smoking, radiation exposure, arsenic in tap water, and even sexually transmitted viral diseases. At this time, there is little available evidence that any of these factors contribute directly to an increased risk.

The fact remains that the majority of prostate cancers have no single, identifiable risk factor that can be pinpointed as a definitive cause. What's a man to do? You can't change your family history or your heritage. But you can change to a low-fat diet, watch your weight, and get plenty of exercise. These are lifestyle changes that will impact far more than your prostate health!

Finally, be cautious of claims that super-high doses of certain vitamins or herbs will stave off prostate cancer or prevent its return. In fact, excessive amounts of many of these supplements can be dangerous, especially if taken over a prolonged period. Common sense—rather than uncommon measures—should be the yardstick used for minimizing your prostate cancer risk.

My Notes

"Initial Questions That I Have"
(Things I just don't understand yet!)

Prevention?

Can prostate cancer be prevented? No, not yet, and maybe never. But we can certainly minimize a number of risk factors for the disease, especially with a low fat, high fruit and vegetable diet, and plenty of exercise.

Beyond these important self-help measures, there are also some promising research initiatives that may bring us closer to the elusive goal of prevention. Two large-scale clinical trials are now taking place. The Prostate Cancer Prevention Trial is testing whether the drug finasteride (Proscar®), proven to be beneficial for the noncancerous prostate condition called benign prostatic hyperplasia (BPH), can also minimize the risk of prostate cancer. (See page 23.)

Similarly, the Selenium and Vitamin E Cancer Prevention Trial (SELECT Trial) is evaluating the preventive benefits of these two dietary supplements. (See page 24.)

A number of researchers are also focusing on modifying dietary and lifestyle factors such as consuming less red meat, eating more fish, and getting more exercise. Other researchers are developing "cancer vaccines" that may have the same revolutionary success as the polio vaccine of yesteryear and the measles vaccine of today.

For now, though, there is no sure-fire way to actually *prevent* prostate cancer. Someday, maybe. But, unfortunately, not yet today.

Exercise

Studies have shown that regular exercise—even 30 minutes, 2 to 3 times a week—can dramatically reduce a person's risk of a number of cancers, including prostate cancer. Additional benefits of exercise include increased lung capacity, muscle strength and greater energy levels. You'll feel more in control, have higher self-esteem, and experience less anxiety and depression. While there will be times during your treatment and recovery when it may be difficult for you to exercise, even a minimal exercise schedule can be tailored to your individual needs.

Some researchers believe that as many as one-third of all prostate cancer cases could be related to lack of exercise and a poor diet—highly preventable risk factors! And yet almost two-thirds of American adults remain inactive, despite the long list of well-known health benefits.

Exercise is a healthy choice to pursue for many reasons, not the least of which is the possibility of reducing your prostate cancer risk.

Diet

As mentioned earlier, a growing number of demographic studies are linking low fat diets to a lower risk of prostate (and other) cancers. While more conclusive studies are needed, the anecdotal evidence is hard to ignore. As diets in Asian countries become more "Westernized" with higher fat content, the incidence of prostate cancer appears to be increasing. The same holds true for first- and second-generation Asian immigrants to the United States, who have a greater risk of developing prostate cancer the longer they have been exposed to the "dietary side effects" of our culture.

Asian diets tend to include more fish than American diets, but they also include more soy and tofu. Do these foods play a role in preventing cancer? Some studies suggest that a diet that regularly includes cooked tomato-based foods may help protect men from prostate cancer.

Other studies have found that diets with high concentrations of fish, especially salmon, herring and mackerel, may have a protective effect against prostate cancer. This may be due in part to a lower consumption of red meat and/or a higher consumption of fruits and vegetables. (Are fish eaters more nutrition-conscious?) Or maybe it is the higher concentration of the fatty acids found in these fish.

Who knows which of these factors, if any, play a role, but it certainly can't hurt to vary your diet a little. You may even enjoy the change!

Finasteride:
The Prostate Cancer Prevention Trial

Good news. A major clinical trial is now under way—The Prostate Cancer Prevention Trial—to see whether the drug finasteride (Proscar®) will reduce the incidence of prostate cancer in men over 55. The seven-year trial, which will end in 2004, will include more than 18,000 men.

Finasteride is currently used to treat a noncancerous condition called benign prostatic hyperplasia (BPH) that causes enlargement of the prostate, as well as prostate cancer. Specifically, finasteride reduces levels of a male hormone called dihydroxytestosterone (DHT), an important compound involved in prostate growth (both normal and abnormal). Since DHT plays a key role in benign (non-cancerous) prostate enlargement, researchers believe that it might also influence the development of prostate cancer.

Researchers involved in the Prostate Cancer Prevention Trial will also be evaluating side effects that finasteride might have on the sexual and urinary functions of men, as well as any other quality-of-life factors that might be impacted.

One note of caution: finasteride may reduce PSA levels by about 50 percent during treatment, thus masking the true PSA level. This may be due to a reduction in the size of the prostate because of the treatment or because the treatment is acting effectively against a potential cancer.

Selenium and Vitamin E: The SELECT Trial

Another major clinical trial will attempt to determine whether two dietary supplements—selenium and vitamin E—can help protect against prostate cancer. The Selenium and Vitamin E Cancer Prevention Trial (SELECT Trial) began enrolling patients in July 2001. It will eventually enroll more than 32,000 men at 400 study sites in the United States, Puerto Rico and Canada.

Selenium was included in the SELECT Trial based on the findings of an earlier decade-long study of patients with skin cancer. During that trial, the researchers noticed that the trace element selenium seemed to have a preventive effect on a number of cancers, including those of the prostate, lung and colorectum. (Unfortunately, selenium did not affect the incidence of skin cancer, as was originally hoped.)

The usual recommended dose for selenium in prostate cancer prevention is 200 mcg per day. Selenium is a trace element that is present in vegetables and grain grown in selenium-rich soil, as well as in other foods, especially fish. However, it would be difficult to consume enough foods on a daily basis to meet the 200 mcg per day recommendation. Therefore, the supplement appears to be necessary.

Do not become overzealous with selenium consumption. Sometimes more is not better. Large amounts may become toxic, resulting in nausea, vomiting, hair and tooth loss, and nail damage.

Similarly, another study involving more than 29,000 Finnish male smokers found that participants taking moderate vitamin E supplements had a substantially reduced incidence of prostate cancer. In fact, the vitamin E group had 32 percent fewer prostate cancer incidences and 41 percent fewer prostate cancer deaths compared with men who did not take the supplement.

(It should be noted that vitamin E may interfere with blood clotting. Therefore, stop taking it one week before any surgical procedure or biopsy.)

The mechanisms by which selenium and vitamin E may reduce prostate cancer risk are not clear. Both are antioxidants, which prevent carcinogens from damaging DNA. Some researchers believe they may inhibit the multiplication of prostate cancer cells. Others think they somehow stimulate the immune system or alter the levels of sex hormones. More studies are clearly needed, and the SELECT Trial is an important step in the right direction.

Those who are interested in learning more about the SELECT Trial can call the National Cancer Institute's Cancer Information Service at 1-800-4CANCER (1-800-422-6237). In Canada, you can call the Canadian Cancer Society's Cancer Information Service at 1-888-939-3333.

Preventing Cancer with Vitamins and Minerals

Studies have shown that more than half of U.S. adults over the age of 65 are taking a wide range of vitamins with the specific aim of *preventing* cancer, (as are a quarter of those aged 55 to 64). However, while eating plenty of fresh fruits and vegetables has been shown in several studies to possibly lower the risk of developing cancer, there is no convincing evidence that taking just vitamin and mineral supplements provides the same benefit. Neither approach is definitive.

There is little doubt that some dietary supplements, when taken in appropriate doses, can provide healthy benefits. The role they might play in preventing cancer, however, has not been sufficiently researched.

Garlic is a great example. Substances found in garlic have been shown to fight cancer in a test tube but, so far, there is no significant evidence that they can do the same in humans. Yet, how many ads for garlic have you seen on TV, in newspapers, magazines, and so on? Are these claims substantiated? We wish they were, but as of today, they are not.

Soy products have received much attention in the last decade as having "protective" effects against many cancers. The fat in soy is unsaturated and therefore tends to lower cholesterol. Soy is also rich in omega-3 fatty acids, which makes fish oil very healthy. Soy also provides fiber, vitamins and minerals such as folate, iron and zinc.

Isoflavones are antioxidants that neutralize harmful molecules produced by normal metabolism. Soy products contain significant levels of isoflavones and thus may protect against cancer. There are more than 4,000 naturally occurring flavonoids. These compounds are found in fruits, nuts, seeds, vegetables and some teas.

Lycopene, a phytochemical that occurs naturally in tomatoes and other fruits, has been demonstrated to reduce the risk of developing prostate cancer. Lycopene supplements are available, but natural sources appear to be better. The best sources of lycopenes are cooked tomatoes, tomato sauce, grapefruit, cabbage, red pepper, strawberries and guava.

Vitamin E may act in conjunction with selenium to provide an antioxidant effect. Recent studies have demonstrated that taking 75 i.u. (international units) of vitamin E daily reduces the risk of developing prostate cancer by 30 percent. The best natural sources of vitamin E are almonds and fruit sugar.

Vitamin D has been shown to have a protective effect against developing prostate cancer. Large doses of calcium (exceeding 2,000 mg/day) may increase the risk of developing prostate cancer, perhaps by inhibiting the body's own production of vitamin D, although fructose seems to counteract this. More research is needed to clarify these interactions.

Most vitamin and mineral supplements are not harmful if taken in appropriate doses—and many may certainly have some benefit. But broad claims that a specific vitamin or mineral supplement can single-handedly prevent cancer from occurring are clearly unsubstantiated.

Furthermore, there is real concern that excessive doses of many of these supplements could, in fact, be harmful. For example, vitamin

A has been linked to an increased risk of stomach cancer, and questions have been raised about the interaction of St. John's Wort with certain medicines.

Some supplements may skew the results of laboratory tests. Others may alter bleeding times—an important consideration if you are about to undergo surgery. Be sure to disclose to your physician any supplements (such as vitamin E) that you are taking on a regular basis.

Cancer Vaccines

Some pioneering cancer researchers are currently working to develop vaccines that will encourage the body's immune system to recognize cancer cells, just as traditional vaccines for mumps and measles target those infectious diseases.

Vaccines work by exposing your body's immune system to a weakened version of the specific disease. This then stimulates your immune system to produce *antibodies* to fight the unwelcome invaders. Once your body has produced antibodies for a specific disease, it can remember how to recognize them in the future. In terms of cancer, these antibodies may destroy any cancer cells that develop, or at least slow their growth.

The manufacture of vaccines against specific cancers is a very promising avenue of cancer research. Such vaccines could be used either as preventive treatments to stop people from actually getting cancer, or could be used together with traditional cancer-fighting treatments (surgery, radiation, chemotherapy) to target existing or recurrent tumors.

While the practical use of vaccines to prevent and treat cancer may still be years away, dramatic advances in our understanding of the human genetic code could move that timetable up significantly.

Risk Reduction

While cancer cannot be "prevented," your risk for the disease or its recurrence may well be minimized. Significant risk *reduction*, rather than prevention, is an achievable goal. And *major* risk reduction is certainly within your personal capability. Researchers are doing their part and making remarkable strides. So can you!

Prevention?

My Notes

"My Personal Risk Factors"
(Which ones can I minimize?)

Screening Techniques

Early detection for prostate cancer is the key to having many more treatment options at your disposal—and a better chance for an excellent outcome. Regular prostate cancer screening is the best way to do this.

Several risk factors increase a man's chances of developing prostate cancer. These factors must be taken into consideration when your doctor recommends screening. Age is the most common risk factor, with the majority of prostate cancer cases being diagnosed in men age 55 and older.

Other risk factors for prostate cancer include family history and race. Men who have a father, brother, son, uncle or cousin with prostate cancer have a greater chance of developing prostate cancer. African-American men have the highest rate of prostate cancer, while Asian-American men have much lower rates.

Even without these risk factors, however, you should strongly consider annual screening for prostate cancer that includes a digital rectal exam by a physician and a blood test to check for elevated levels of prostate-specific antigen (PSA) beginning at age 50. African-American men and men with a family history of prostate cancer should begin regular screening at age 40.

Digital Rectal Exam

A digital rectal exam (DRE) is a physical exam in which your doctor feels for abnormalities in the prostate gland. Your doctor will insert a lubricated, gloved finger into the rectum and feel the prostate gland through the rectal wall to check for enlargement, bumps or abnormal areas. This is a fast procedure and minimally uncomfortable.

Although the digital rectal exam has been used for many years, it is not perfect because it is based on the skill and subjective judgment of the individual physician. While still an important screening tool, it should be done in conjunction with a PSA test.

Prostate-Specific Antigen (PSA)

The prostate-specific antigen (PSA) test measures the level of PSA in the blood. PSA is a protein produced by the cells of the prostate gland. When the prostate gland enlarges, or when prostate cancer is present, PSA levels in the blood tend to rise. Unfortunately, PSA levels alone do not give doctors enough information to distinguish between benign prostate conditions and cancer.

The PSA level that is considered normal for an average older man ranges from 0 to 4 ng/ml (nanograms/milliliter). A PSA level of 4 to 10 ng/ml requires further evaluation; levels above 10 ng/ml are considered highly suspicious.

The higher the PSA level, the more likely it is that cancer is present. However, there could be other possible reasons for an elevated PSA level. These include: benign prostate enlargement, inflammation, infection, age, race, certain medications, and ejaculation within 24 hours prior to the test.

On the other hand, if you currently have prostate cancer and are being treated with hormone therapy, you should have a low PSA reading during, or immediately after, treatment. This can be an indication that the treatment is working, as well as a measure of PSA activity in the body.

Other Screening Tests

If the results of either a digital rectal exam or a PSA test are abnormal, your doctor may recommend further evaluation. This may include the following: a sonogram of the prostate gland (transrectal ultrasonography), another blood test to confirm a PSA elevation, or a biopsy. In some situations, your physician may consider a course of antibiotics, followed by another check of your PSA.

Transrectal ultrasonography is a sonogram that uses sound waves to create a two-dimensional image of the prostate gland. A small probe is inserted into the rectum to take the images. Transrectal ultrasonography is generally used as an aid to prostate biopsy and not specifically as a screening tool.

Prostatic acid phosphatase (PAP) is an enzyme that is normally present only in small amounts in the blood. It may be found at higher levels in some patients with prostate cancer. However, PAP levels may also be elevated in patients who have certain benign prostatic conditions. (This test is rarely used today.)

Biopsy is the only definitive way to diagnose prostate cancer. In a biopsy, a thin needle, guided by ultrasound, is used to remove samples of prostate tissue. These samples are then checked under a microscope for cancerous cells.

False Positive/False Negative Results

Unfortunately, we don't have a foolproof screening test for prostate cancer. A digital rectal exam is still subject to the interpretive skills of the physician performing it; a PSA test can sometimes provide "false positive" or "false negative" results.

"False positive" test results occur when the PSA level is elevated, but no cancer is actually present. False positives may lead to unnecessary additional testing, with significant financial costs—not to mention anxiety for you and your family.

"False negative" results occur when the PSA level is in the normal range even though prostate cancer is actually present. Most prostate cancers are slow-growing and therefore subsequent tests should indicate a trend so that appropriate treatment can be undertaken.

"I Flunked My PSA!"

Because such false positive and false negative results with PSA do occur, it is important for prostate cancer screening to take place on an *ongoing* basis to track the *trend* of PSA levels.

New Screening Techniques

Because of the problems of false positive and false negative PSA values, researchers are trying to develop better methods of using PSA to screen for prostate cancer. Some of these new techniques include:

Free PSA – An important new PSA screening test such as Hybritech® measures the percent of "free PSA" in the body, which helps the physician distinguish between prostate cancer and non-cancerous prostate disease. PSA circulates in the blood in two forms: free, or attached to a protein molecule. With benign prostate conditions, there is more "free" PSA, while cancer produces more of the "attached" form. (See page 35.)

PSA velocity – PSA velocity is a measure of changes in PSA levels over time. A sharp rise in the PSA level raises the suspicion of cancer.

Age-adjusted PSA – Age is a factor that can cause increasing PSA levels. For this reason, some doctors use "age-adjusted" PSA levels to determine when further diagnostic tests are needed. For example, men younger than age 50 should have a PSA level below 2.5 ng/ml, while a PSA level up to 6.5 ng/ml might be considered normal for men in their 70s. There is some disagreement among doctors about the accuracy and usefulness of age-adjusted PSA levels, although the vast majority of urologists accept this diagnostic technology.

PSA density – PSA density compares the PSA level to the size and weight of the prostate. In other words, an elevated PSA might not arouse suspicion in a man with a very large prostate. The use of PSA density to interpret PSA results is controversial because cancer might be overlooked in a man with an enlarged prostate gland.

PROSTATE CANCER
Free-to-total PSA*

PSA	Probability of Cancer
2 ng/mL	1%
2-4 ng/mL	15%
4-10 ng/mL	25%
>10 ng/mL	>50%

% FPSA	Probability of Cancer
0-10%	56%
10-15%	28%
15-20%	20%
20-25%	16%
>25%	8%

*Men with non-suspicious DRE results, regardless of patient age.

Brawer MK. Prostate-specific antigen: Current status. *CA Cancer J Clin*. 1999;49(5):264-281.

It should be noted that PSA velocity, age-adjusted PSA and PSA density are not widely utilized in clinical practice. However, the measure of free PSA appears to be a useful screening tool, especially for patients with PSA values between 4 to 10 ng/ml.

Minority Screening

Prostate cancer screening levels among minority groups in the United States have historically been significantly lower than those for Caucasians. Different studies have blamed unequal access to healthcare facilities, income and educational disparities, cultural biases, and even a lingering distrust of the medical establishment.

Quite simply, the direct result of lower screening levels is unacceptably higher death rates. Yet studies have shown that if patients of any racial or ethnic background are given equal screening and treatment opportunities, similar survival rates will result.

Nonetheless, the fact remains that screening rates for minority groups are, in general, far too low. This is especially crucial for diseases such as prostate cancer that strike African Americans at disproportionately higher levels.

In 1970, racial and ethnic minority groups accounted for 16 percent of the U.S. population. By 2050 they will comprise nearly half of the population. By the year 2010 Hispanics will surpass African Americans as the largest U.S. racial or ethnic group. By the year 2050, 23 percent of the entire U.S. population is expected to be Hispanic. Based on sheer numbers alone, greater research into minority screening and treatment programs should become an urgent priority.

For more information on screening programs in your community, ask your healthcare provider or call the Cancer Information Service at 1-800-4CANCER. Prostate cancer is a highly treatable disease, especially if caught early. That makes it even more tragic when important screening opportunities are not provided to those most in need.

TABLE I
Screening Guidelines for Prostate Cancer

Under Age 50:
Screening Recommendation - PSA blood test and digital rectal exam (DRE) are offered to men age 40 to 50 at high risk for prostate cancer after being informed about the controversy surrounding risks and benefits.

You may be at high risk if:

- You have a family history of prostate cancer (father, brother, son, uncle, cousin), particularly if diagnosed before age 50.
- You have had a previous biopsy with a pathologic diagnosis of prostatic intraepithelial neoplasia.
- You have a history of fluctuating PSA levels (even if less than 4 ng/ml).
- You are an African-American male.

Age 50 to 70:
Screening Recommendation – It is suggested that the option of annual screening be offered to men age 50 to 70 after they have been informed of the controversy surrounding risks and benefits.

Over Age 70:
We do not recommend screening because most prostate cancers that might lead to death occur before age 70. Men who develop prostate cancer over age 70 will most likely not be affected by this disease depending on their life expectancy.

All males are at high risk if they have:

- A family history of prostate cancer (father, brother, son, uncle, cousin), particularly if diagnosed before age 50.
- A previous biopsy with a pathologic diagnosis of prostatic intraepithelial neoplasia.
- A history of fluctuating PSA levels (even if less than 4 ng/ml).
- African-American ancestry.

Benign (Non-Cancerous) Prostate Conditions

As men age, the risk increases for both benign (non-cancerous) prostate conditions and for prostate cancer. The most common non-cancerous prostate conditions are *benign prostatic hyperplasia (BPH), prostatitis,* and *prostatic intraepithelial neoplasia (PIN).*

Benign prostatic hyperplasia (BPH) is the abnormal growth of benign (non-cancerous) prostate cells. In BPH, the prostate grows larger and larger, pressing against the urethra and interfering with the normal flow of urine.

More than half of all men in the United States between the ages of 60 and 70, and as many as 90 percent of men between the ages of 70 and 90, have symptoms of BPH. These symptoms include frequency, urgency, frequent nighttime urination, decreased stream strength, and occasional urinary retention (requiring a catheter for emptying the bladder.)

Prostatitis is a condition in which the prostate becomes infected or inflamed. This may cause swelling of the prostate gland and pressure against the urethra and bladder. This can impede the flow of urine and possibly cause a burning sensation during urination.

Prostatic intraepithelial neoplasia (PIN) is characterized by abnormal cellular growth and proliferation within the prostate ducts and glands. PIN has no symptoms. It coexists with prostate cancer in more than 85 percent of cases. PIN may develop years before prostate cancer. It is most often discovered during a biopsy resulting from an elevated PSA, or when a procedure is being performed for relief of the symptoms of BPH.

There is no evidence that either BPH or prostatitis cause cancer. However, it is possible for a man to have one or both of these conditions, and prostate cancer as well. PIN, by contrast, while not a cancer, is considered by most to be a precursor to the disease.

The Prostate, Lung, Colorectal, and Ovarian Cancer Screening Trial

The Prostate, Lung, Colorectal, and Ovarian Cancer Screening Trial, or PLCO Trial, is a major clinical trial being sponsored by the National Cancer Institute. It will eventually enroll up to 150,000 men and women to evaluate the effectiveness of certain cancer screening tests.

Different screening tests are being studied for each of these four types of cancer. For prostate cancer, the effectiveness of regular screening with a digital rectal exam (DRE) and PSA test will be evaluated to determine their impact on reducing mortality from the disease. Men participating in the PLCO Trial will be randomized to have either annual DRE and PSA screening over a three-year period, or undergo standard healthcare from their physicians (the control group).

If you are interested in participating in the PLCO Trial, you can call the National Cancer Institute's Cancer Information Service at 1–800–4CANCER. Information about the PLCO Trial can also be found on the Internet at: http://dcp.nci.nih.gov/plco/default.html.

PART II:

Diagnosis and Treatment

A Diagnosis of Cancer: What Does It Mean?

"I am so sorry to tell you that you have cancer." It is difficult to imagine more earth-shattering words. In an instant, your world turns upside down.

How can you possibly absorb such news? Some people express shock, others confusion. Some lash out and become angry, others withdraw and go into denial. Most are in a state of uncertainty and fear.

All of these reactions are totally normal. In fact, if you do not express one of these reactions, your physician may become worried about how you are coping.

That's the bad news. The good news is that there are very effective treatment options available today that will enable you to live a long and prosperous life. Yes, you will have some bumps in the road, but you can—*and will*—get over those.

From here on, it is very important that you try to understand everything you can about your diagnosis. At what stage was your cancer caught? What treatment options are available? What side effects might result from those treatments?

Always remember that you are not alone! Whether it's your spouse or significant other, family members, close friends, and/or your healthcare team—at a time like this you will find how blessed you are to have these special people who will now support you. They will become an extraordinary source of encouragement.

Keep in mind that cancer doesn't just strike *you*—it affects your loved ones as well. While it may be difficult to "let others do for you," it's very important for them to feel as though they can help you in your time of need. On the other hand, don't let them overwhelm you. Be strong. They need that from you, as they are hurting as well.

If you do not have anyone close to you, there are many support groups, community organizations, church programs, and other resources that can be of immense assistance. Contact them. Don't hesitate to ask for help and support. That is what they are there for—and they want to help. It will make them feel good that you called.

Recognizing Symptoms

Prostate cancer most often has no symptoms until it has become advanced. In fact, most prostate cancer patients are asymptomatic (without symptoms) and may remain so for a long period of time. This is why screening is important to help diagnose the disease in its earliest stages. Some men, however, do experience some symptoms that may indicate prostate cancer. These include:

- A need to urinate frequently, especially at night;
- Difficulty starting or stopping urinary flow;
- Weak or interrupted flow of urine;
- Painful or burning urination;
- Difficulty in achieving an erection;
- Painful ejaculation;
- Blood in the urine or semen;
- Inability to urinate; or,
- Frequent pain or stiffness in the lower back, hips & upper thighs.

The above symptoms may be caused by a variety of conditions, and if you are experiencing any of them, do not become alarmed. As men age, their prostate may grow bigger and block the flow of urine or interfere with normal sexual function. Often these are the result of non-cancerous conditions (BPH, prostatitis) that certainly do not represent cancer but may require treatment with medicines or surgery. It is therefore important to check with your doctor if you are experiencing any of these symptoms.

Stages of Prostate Cancer

If cancer is found in the prostate, the doctor will "stage" the disease to determine whether the cancer has spread and, if so, what other parts of the body are affected. This is extremely important for determining the best treatment option for you.

The following stages are used for prostate cancer:

Stage I or Stage A – The cancer cannot be felt during a rectal exam. It may be found incidentally when surgery is done for another reason, usually for benign prostatic hyperplasia (BPH). There is no evidence that the cancer has spread outside the prostate.

Stage II or Stage B – The tumor can be felt during a rectal exam. There is no evidence that the cancer has spread outside the prostate.

Stage III or Stage C – The cancer has spread locally outside the prostate to nearby tissues. There is no evidence of distant (metastatic) disease.

Stage IV or Stage D – The cancer has spread to lymph nodes, bones or to other parts of the body.

Prostate cancer can also be classified by T stages as follows:

T1 – The tumor cannot be felt during a digital rectal exam, but cancer cells are found in a prostate biopsy or prostatectomy specimen. T1 cancers can be subdivided as: *T1a* (less than 5 percent of the removed tissue is cancerous); *T1b* (more than 5 percent of the removed tissue is cancerous); or *T1c* (the cancer is found as a result of PSA screening).

T2 – The tumor can be felt during a digital rectal exam, but the cancer appears to be confined to the prostate gland. T2 cancers can be subdivided as: *T2a* (the tumor involves only one side of the prostate); or *T2b* (the tumor involves both sides of the prostate).

T3 – The cancer has spread to the connective tissue next to the prostate or to the seminal vesicles, but does not involve any other organs. T3 cancers can be divided as: *T3a* (the cancer has spread outside the prostate but does not involve the seminal vesicles); or *T3b* (the cancer has spread to the seminal vesicles).

T4 – The cancer has spread to tissues beyond the prostate and seminal vesicles.

Refer to Appendix I (page 89) for detailed illustrations of the stages of prostate cancer.

The Gleason Score

When a prostate biopsy is done, the pathologist will use various measures to determine whether cancer is present and, if so, how aggressive the cancer may be. One of the most useful measures is the Gleason score. Gleason scores range from 2 to 10. In general, a score of 2 to 4 indicates low aggressiveness for the cancer, and a score of 5 to 6 indicates moderate aggressiveness. A score of 7 to 10 signifies a more aggressive tumor.

Gleason scores are based on how the patterns of cells (differentiation) look under a microscope. Prostate cancer cells are more disorganized and form abnormal patterns (are poorly differentiated) compared with normal cells. This may be an indication that they will be more aggressive. The pathologist assigns a grade to these patterns, with a higher score indicating a more aggressive cancer. The Gleason score is just one of the ways in which your doctor assesses the best treatment options for your cancer.

Family and Friends are Impacted Too

Unfortunately, you are not the only one impacted by the diagnosis of prostate cancer. Your family and close friends are also affected. They have to deal with their own feelings as well as be sensitive to

A Diagnosis of Cancer

yours throughout treatment and recovery.

Often, family members absorb the brunt of a cancer patient's anger and frustration. They in turn may even lash back, expressing anger, hurt or frustration at their own powerlessness over the situation you are facing.

Remember that your family and close friends will be your most valuable source of support. They hopefully know when to simply listen, or when to encourage feelings to be shared. They can help make sure that the right questions are asked, or that questions are asked at all. And they can help you understand the incredible amount of new information now consuming your life.

This "second set of ears" can be extremely important. Studies have shown that the information retained by a patient after a cancer diagnosis is surprisingly incomplete. One study found that only 60 percent correctly recalled what their treatment entailed; 41 percent could not list a single major treatment risk; and only 27 percent could name one treatment alternative.

Even when physicians are conscientious in communicating specific details regarding treatment and prognosis, patients often do not remember what was said. Hospital patients in general typically remember just over 50 percent of the information they receive from doctors about their diagnosis and treatment. This figure drops to less than 25 percent for cancer patients. Distressing information may raise your anxiety level and significantly reduce your ability to remember details.

Hearing unexpected and unwanted information causes many people to focus on a particular word or sentence while the doctor keeps talking. **No problem.** Simply have it repeated. Or better yet, bring someone with you to all of your medical appointments and afterward discuss with them the treatment options that have been presented to you by your physician.

It can be extremely helpful to bring a tape recorder so that you can listen in the privacy of your home to your doctor's explanation—over and over again, as many times as necessary. (Don't be surprised at how much you missed!)

Coping with cancer can be extremely challenging, but it doesn't have to be overwhelming—and it doesn't have to be undertaken alone.

Speak Up During Doctor Visits

Studies have shown that as many as three-quarters of cancer patients' questions are *not* asked during medical appointments. Why? Fear of humiliation in front of the doctor is the most commonly cited reason. You may worry that your doctor will misunderstand your motivation for questioning, or think that you are second-guessing his or her judgment. And with so much going on, you may not want to risk ruining your relationship with your doctor.

Further, you may feel urgency about the amount of time you are taking from your doctor's "needier" patients. Feeling hurried obviously interferes with your ability to gather thoughts and clearly articulate questions.

Forget about hurting your doctor's feelings with questions, or taking up too much of his or her time. It is very important to keep in mind that *you're* the one with cancer. *You're* the one with the ultimate authority to make any treatment decisions. Your doctor is only a professional guide through *your* treatment and recovery.

That means *you* are ultimately responsible for adequately communicating to your doctor your concerns and needs, and to mention any other treatments that you are considering. This is especially true with complementary and alternative therapies such as herbs, dietary supplements, megadoses of vitamins, and other measures.

About three-quarters of cancer patients use alternative therapies such as acupuncture, herbs, prayer or nutritional supplements, but only a third of these patients disclose their use of such treatments to their doctors. This lack of disclosure can sometimes lead to complications.

For example, some herbal supplements can skew the results of laboratory tests; some may increase the tendency to bleed during surgery; still others may cause side effects that are incorrectly attributed to an effective conventional treatment. **Talk to your doctor!**

Talking to Your Kids

What if you have children, especially young ones? Or even grandchildren? How do you tell *them* about your cancer? This is difficult enough with adult family members and friends, but it can be especially disconcerting with children.

The reason for such difficulties is a fear of the questions the children may ask, particularly about the possibility of death. You may be concerned about causing too much anxiety and stress for your children, or you may think they will not understand. You want to protect them. That is a **totally normal** concern.

Such assumptions may make a difficult situation even worse for a child. Experts agree that communication is *essential* for children to be able to cope with the illness of a parent. So what should you tell the kids? And when?

Tell children about your illness as soon as possible. Children as young as four and five will feel the tension in the home. When there's a delay, or if it's kept a family secret, they will build up resentment and quite possibly "imagine the worst."

But how to begin? The approach depends partly on each child's age and your personal relationship with them. Be as honest as possible, phrasing the discussion in terms of "love and hopefulness." Watch how they *individually* respond to what you are saying and continue your talk accordingly. Every child (and every adult, for that matter) will react and cope in their own unique way.

Reassure them that the cancer is not contagious and is not due to anything they did. (This is especially important for younger children.) Tell them that they will continue to be cared for no matter how family routines may temporarily be disrupted.

Even when the prognosis is poor, it is still possible to speak truthfully and with hope. For example, you might say: "Some people die from cancer, but many get better. I'm working very hard to be one of the people who gets better."

Along with providing honesty and reassurance to your children, watch for signs that they are not coping well, including significant changes in mood or personality, decreased appetite, withdrawal from friends and family, a drop in grades, or behavioral problems at school.

Second Opinions

Five words about second opinions—*"Don't hesitate to get one!"* This is especially true with prostate cancer because of the many treatment options available to you. If you feel at all uncomfortable with your doctor, if you consistently do not understand what is being recommended, or if you believe there are treatment options that are not being offered, you have the right—the obligation—to ask for a second opinion. Switch doctors if you feel the need.

Second opinions are often pursued for reasons far beyond the risk of misdiagnosis. Doctors sometimes perform procedures that they feel more comfortable with, rather than basing treatment decisions on the medical evidence available.

Even when there are no treatment alternatives to sort out, and no problems exist between you and your doctor, a second opinion can offer a fresh perspective. Maybe it can confirm a diagnosis or reinforce the wisdom of a course of treatment, and thus ease any doubts that you, or your family, may have. If you sense reluctance from your doctor about getting a second opinion, that may be all the more reason to get one. Remember, your physician works for *you*.

My Notes

"Questions To Ask My Doctor"
(To be answered <u>during</u> my appointment!)

Understanding Your Treatment Options

The primary treatment strategies for prostate cancer have remained relatively consistent—watchful waiting, surgery, radiation therapy and hormonal therapy—and refinements in these techniques have made each of them *much* more effective. The relatively new option of cryosurgery is also available, as are a number of extremely promising new treatments now being evaluated in large-scale clinical trials.

While you should be given treatment options by your doctor, all of the final decisions will be left up to you. Keep this in mind—you can make no wrong choice in your decision. Whatever option you might choose, at whatever stage of treatment, is the **right decision** for *you.*

Your individual situation will direct your best options for treatment. **Your choice is extremely important** and should be discussed at length with your doctor. This may be the time to consider a second opinion just to be sure that the treatment option you choose is indeed the most appropriate for you.

Watchful Waiting

Prostate cancer, fortunately, tends to be a slow-growing cancer. As such, "watchful waiting" may be an appropriate treatment option for some men, especially if they are older and the cancer is found at an early stage (Gleason score of 2 to 4). Watchful waiting means that no treatment will be undertaken at this time. There will be close monitoring of your condition and treatment may eventually be recommended. But not now.

Watchful waiting may also be advised for men with other medical problems for whom the risks and side effects of surgery, radiation therapy, or hormonal therapy outweigh their possible benefits.

The chief advantage of watchful waiting is no immediate side effects or complications. However, an *essential* part of watchful waiting is regular monitoring to make sure that the disease is not progressing. The anxiety of repeated examinations, blood tests and other evaluation techniques may take a toll on you and your loved ones. If you feel you cannot cope with such frequent examinations and waiting for their results, you should consider additional therapy. (In one study, 50 percent of the men who initially chose watchful waiting switched to more aggressive treatments within two years due to anxiety.)

An important clinical study, the Prostate Cancer Outcomes Study or PCOS (see page 64), is now under way to better assess the value of watchful waiting in men with early stage prostate cancer, as well as to decide when additional treatment may become necessary.

Side Effects of Watchful Waiting

Although some men choose watchful waiting to avoid the side effects of surgery, radiation and other treatments, this choice may involve a considerable risk. Watchful waiting may reduce the chance of controlling the disease before it spreads. In addition, older men should keep in mind that it may be harder to tolerate surgery and radiation therapy as they age.

Some men may decide against watchful waiting because they feel they would be uncomfortable living with an untreated cancer, even one that appears to be growing slowly or perhaps not at all. Keep in mind that an initial decision for watchful waiting can always be changed to more aggressive treatment as your personal circumstances change—medical, emotional or otherwise. It is *your* decision and a different treatment approach is *always* available.

Surgery

Surgery remains the most common treatment for early stage prostate cancer. *Radical prostatectomy* is the removal of the prostate and some of the tissues around it. The doctor may do the surgery by cutting into the space between the scrotum and the anus (the perineum) in an operation called a *perineal prostatectomy,* or by an incision in the lower abdomen in an operation called a *retropubic prostatectomy.*

In some cases, the doctor can use a technique known as a *nerve-sparing prostatectomy*, which attempts to save the nerves that control erection. Men with large tumors or tumors that are very close to the nerves may not be able to have this type of surgery.

Transurethral resection of the prostate (TURP) uses an instrument inserted through the penis to access the prostate through the urethra. This operation is most often done to relieve obstructive symptoms caused by the tumor before other treatments are pursued. (It is also used to relieve symptoms of noncancerous prostatic enlargement.)

Radical prostatectomy is usually done only if there is no evidence that the cancer has spread outside the prostate. Before proceeding with a radical prostatecomy, the surgeon may remove some of the lymph nodes in the pelvis to see if they contain cancer. This is called a *pelvic lymph node dissection*. If the lymph nodes contain considerable cancer, your surgeon may decide not to continue with the prostatectomy. Unfortunately, you cannot know beforehand if the procedure will be performed. This can only be decided at the time of surgery, while you are under anesthesia.

The chief benefit of radical prostatectomy is that it surgically "stages" the cancer. The patient can get a much better picture of his prognosis than with any non-surgical treatments. If the cancer is truly localized, radical prostatectomy can cure the patient. However, this procedure's ability to reveal something definitive about your staging and prognosis must be weighed against the potential side effects of the operation.

With radical prostatectomy there is a significant risk of impotence and incontinence. Surgery must therefore be compared to the potential effectiveness of other viable treatment options. Your physician uses the Gleason score, stage, PSA and other variables to help determine which treatment options are most suited for you. This is an extremely important decision; once again, it is *your* decision.

A recent development in radical prostatectomy is the use of laparoscopic techniques. This new approach may reduce the risk of impotence and incontinence in patients needing the procedure. Less scarring, less blood loss and a significantly shorter recovery time are the cited benefits of this minimally invasive procedure.

Laparoscopic radical prostatectomy is performed through several small incisions in the abdomen. A viewing camera and other instruments are then passed into the abdomen; the surgeon operates while viewing a monitor. The procedure, while FDA-approved, is still considered experimental and data on long-term outcomes is not yet available.

Side Effects of Surgery

Side effects from surgery will vary depending on the type of surgery involved and your own personal circumstances. In the short term, nausea and vomiting from anesthesia may be the most immediate side effects. People who are susceptible to motion sickness, have diabetes, or are obese are more prone to experience postoperative nausea and vomiting. Headaches, generalized body aches and pains, and fatigue are very common and totally normal.

Five to ten percent of patients undergoing a radical prostatectomy may require a blood transfusion during surgery. Most patients will be asked to donate their own blood before the operation in case they require a transfusion. After surgery you will have a urinary catheter for several weeks. The catheter drains urine out of your bladder into a sterile bag. Your nurse or doctor will teach you how to care for it.

You will be given medications to control pain and bladder spasms. You may also need a stool softener so you won't have to strain when going to the bathroom and risk irritating the operative area.

Surgery to remove the prostate may cause significant long-term problems, including *impotence* (the inability to have an unassisted erection), urinary *incontinence* (not being able to control when to urinate), and *urgency* (the feeling of a need to urinate quickly). These are significant side effects that affect many men, often for short periods, but occasionally for life. Not all men experience these side effects, but the risks are high enough that they should be weighed into your treatment decision.

The risk of impotence appears to be age-dependent. Your presurgical ability to achieve an erection is an important predictor of potency following surgery. Younger men and those with no impotency-associated symptoms prior to surgery suffer far less from impotence after surgery than those who have problems prior to surgery.

Men who have a prostatectomy no longer produce semen, so they have *dry orgasms*. While the pleasurable feeling of orgasm remains, no semen is actually ejaculated.

Radiation Therapy

Radiation therapy (also called radiotherapy) uses high-energy x-rays or proton beams to kill cancer cells. Like surgery, radiation therapy is a *local therapy*—it can affect cancer cells only in the treated area. In early stage prostate cancer, radiation can be used instead of surgery, or it may be used after surgery to destroy any cancer cells that may remain in the area. In advanced stages, it may be used for pain control, especially if the cancer has spread to any bones in the body.

Radiation may be directed at the body by a machine (*external radiation*), or it may come from tiny radioactive "seeds" placed inside or near the tumor (*internal* or *implant radiation*, or *brachytherapy*). Some men with prostate cancer receive both external and implant radiation therapy. Men who receive radioactive seeds alone usually have small localized tumors with an acceptable Gleason score (below 7) and a low PSA.

Prior to receiving *external radiation therapy*, a process called a "simulation" will be undertaken by the radiation therapist. This involves identifying the specific areas to be targeted for radiation. The simulation may use x-rays, CT scans or other imaging studies to plan the path of radiation. Small tattoo dots are placed on the body so that the subsequent radiation can be administered accurately to the same area each time.

External radiation therapy is typically given 5 days a week for 7 to 8 weeks. Treatments last only minutes, although travel, waiting time, and talking with the medical staff can add up. Most patients are in and out of the radiation center in less than an hour.

Implant radiation or *brachytherapy* involves the placement of a number of small radioactive "seeds" within the prostate. The procedure takes 1 to 2 hours and is usually performed on an outpatient basis. You will be given a spinal or general anesthetic and the seeds will be implanted using small needles. The surgeon will direct the location of the needles and placement of the seeds via an ultrasound probe inserted into the rectum.

Brachytherapy has the advantage of being able to direct high doses of radiation to specific areas. It is a minimally invasive procedure that appears to be very effective; follow-up studies out to eight years have shown an effectiveness rate equivalent to surgery. A number of studies are ongoing to see if brachytherapy is as effective as surgery in the long-term. It appears that it may well be.

With brachytherapy, there is still a likelihood of impotence, with the risk approaching 25 percent. There is no long-term risk of radiation exposure to yourself or others, but you will be asked to use a condom during the first few months after the procedure to be absolutely safe. In addition, it is recommended that you avoid close and prolonged contact with pregnant women and newborn infants for several months.

Understanding Your Treatment Options

While there are dozens of companies currently manufacturing seeds, only 8 have received certification from the Radiation Therapy Oncology Group (RTOC). These manufacturers are listed in Table II (page 60). Ask your doctor which manufacturer makes the seeds that you may have inserted.

Side Effects of Radiation Therapy

Fatigue is very common during radiation therapy. Your body will use a lot of extra energy over the course of your treatment, and you may feel progressively more tired. Be sure to eat well, get plenty of rest, and sleep or nap as often as you feel the need. It is common for the fatigue to last for 4 to 6 weeks after your treatment has been completed.

Some men may have diarrhea or frequent and uncomfortable urination. In addition, if you are receiving external radiation therapy, it is common for the skin in the treated area to become red, dry and tender. External radiation therapy can also cause hair loss in the treated area. The loss may be temporary or permanent, depending on the dose of radiation as well as your own body's response to the radiation.

Both external and implant radiation therapy may cause impotence in some men, but implant radiation therapy is not as likely to damage the nerves that control erection. Both external and implant radiation therapy may cause mild, temporary incontinence. Long-term incontinence is rare.

It is impossible to predict which side effects you may experience, and to what degree you may experience them. Everyone reacts differently to any therapy, and most patients do not experience all of the side effects mentioned. As with any treatment option, carefully weigh the potential risks and benefits before making your decision. Based on your individual anatomy and other medical conditions, your physician may recommend a particular treatment that could have far fewer side effects.

TABLE II

Brachytherapy Seeds Approved By
The Radiation Therapy Oncology Group

Iodine - 125 Seeds

Nycomed-Amersham model 6702
Nycomed-Amersham model 6711
Best model 2301
International Isotopes/Imagyn Isostar model 12501
North American Scientific/Mentor IoGold model MED3631-A/M
Bebig/UroMed Symmetra model 125.S06

Palladium - 103 Seeds

Theragenics model 200
North American Scientific/Mentor model Med 3633

* Approved as of 10/2001 by the American Association of Physicists in Medicine Radiation Therapy Committee for the Radiation Therapy Oncology Group. Approvals are updated on a frequent basis, therefore other manufacturers may have received an approval after the time of this publication.

Understanding Your Treatment Options

Hormonal Therapy

Hormonal therapy is the use of medications to reduce the hormones that may be stimulating the growth of cancer cells. Hormonal therapy for prostate cancer can take several forms. Male hormones (especially testosterone) are essential to male growth and development, but they can also promote prostate cancer growth when a cancer is present. Ninety-five percent of testosterone is made in the testicles and about 5 percent is made in the adrenal glands.

Hormonal therapies include orchiectomy, LH-RH (luteinizing hormone-releasing hormone) agonists, and antiandrogens.

Orchiectomy is the surgical removal of the testicles, which are the main source of male hormones. This treatment is usually reserved for men with advanced prostate cancer.

Drugs known as *LH-RH agonists* can prevent the testicles from producing testosterone. Examples include *leuprolide (Lupron®)* and *goserelin (Zolodex®)*.

Drugs known as *antiandrogens* can block the action of androgens. Examples include *flutamide (Eulexin®) and bicalutamide (Casodex®)*. Drugs that can prevent the *adrenal glands* from making androgens may also be given. These include *ketoconazole (Nizoral®)*.

After orchiectomy or treatment with an LH-RH agonist, the body no longer gets testosterone from the testicles. However, the adrenal glands still produce small amounts of male hormones. Sometimes, the patient is also given an *antiandrogen*, which blocks the effect of any remaining male hormones. This combination of treatments is known as *complete androgen blockade*.

We do not know for sure whether complete androgen blockade is more effective than orchiectomy or an LH-RH agonist alone. For every trial showing benefit from complete androgen blockade, two others seem to show no benefit.

For advanced prostate cancer, the current consensus in the scientific community is that orchiectomy or an LH-RH agonist alone are sufficient treatments.

Your physician may recommend a course of hormonal therapy prior to surgery or radiation. This occurs most often when the prostate or prostate cancer is very large. The administration of pre-operative hormonal therapy will hopefully shrink the prostate and make the cancer cells more vulnerable so that radiation therapy will have a higher success rate. Concurrent hormonal-radiation therapy is typically offered to patients with locally advanced or high-risk disease (high Gleason score, seminal vesicle involvement, etc.)

Prostate cancer that has spread to other parts of the body can usually be controlled with hormonal therapy for a period of time, often several years. Eventually, however, most prostate cancers continue to grow because they have become resistant to hormonal therapy. When this occurs, hormonal therapy is no longer effective and your doctor may suggest other forms of treatment. You may wish to consider entering a clinical trial of a promising new treatment under study.

Side Effects of Hormonal Therapy

The side effects of hormonal therapy depend largely on the type of treatment. Orchiectomy and LH-RH agonists often cause loss of sexual desire, hot flashes and impotence. When first taken, an LH-RH agonist may worsen your symptoms for a short time, especially if you have advanced cancer. This temporary problem is called a "flare." Gradually, however, the treatment causes a man's testosterone levels to fall. (To prevent a flare, your doctor may prescribe an antiandrogen to be taken for a period of time before the LH-RH agonist.)

Antiandrogens can cause nausea, vomiting, diarrhea, or breast growth and tenderness if used for a prolonged period of time. Men who receive complete androgen blockade may experience more side effects than men who receive a single method of hormonal therapy.

In addition, any method of prolonged hormonal therapy that lowers androgen levels may contribute to significant weakening of the bones, especially in older men (osteoporosis). There are treatments available to greatly reduce the risk of osteoporosis.

Treatment Options: Choosing Between Them

The most difficult choice you will have to make is deciding between the various treatment options that are currently available. Each has advantages and disadvantages. They may all be good options; again, **there is no wrong choice!**

Perhaps more so with prostate cancer than any other type of cancer, significant individual factors must be considered when choosing a treatment plan. These include both the medical characteristics of your cancer (the size and location of the tumor; if it is still localized; its clinical stage), as well as the potential quality of life risks that may follow each choice (impotence, incontinence. etc.).

Your age will also come into play, both in terms of the risk of the potential side effects from aggressive treatments as well as the viability of the "watchful waiting" alternative.

It is therefore extremely important to discuss all of your treatment options with your physician. At this point, you should strongly consider a second opinion if you feel at all uncomfortable with the treatment options that have been presented to you. Don't be timid or embarrassed. Remember, it is *your* body, *your* health—and *your* decision.

New Treatments on the Horizon

Many new treatment options will soon be emerging from ongoing clinical trials. For example, *gene therapy* is a treatment that modifies genes and then reinjects them into your body to fight your cancer.

With gene therapy, researchers are trying to stimulate the body's natural abilities to fight the disease more effectively, or to make the cancer more sensitive to other cancer-fighting treatments.

Another avenue of research is focusing on attacking the *blood vessels* of a tumor rather than the tumor itself. The process by which new blood vessels are formed is called *angiogenesis*. This new cancer-fighting strategy involves the development of *angiogenesis inhibitors*—compounds that act to interrupt the process of tumor blood vessel formation. When tumors are deprived of their blood supply, they starve and go away.

Cryosurgery, sometimes called *cryoablation,* is under study as an alternative to surgery and radiation therapy. With cryosurgery, the doctor tries to avoid damaging healthy tissues by placing an instrument known as a cryoprobe in direct contact with the tumor in order to freeze it. The extreme cold destroys the cancer cells.

Some researchers are studying the effectiveness of *chemotherapy* and *biological therapy* for men whose prostate cancers are not responding to hormonal therapy. Other researchers are exploring new treatment schedules and combinations. For example, they are studying the usefulness of hormonal therapy before primary therapy (surgery or radiation) to shrink large tumors and make them more responsive to subsequent treatment.

There are many other promising research alternatives. If your disease is more advanced, we urge you to consider enrolling in a clinical trial to test one of these potentially revolutionary new treatment options. Ask your doctor if there are any clinical trials that may be appropriate for you.

The Prostate Cancer Outcomes Study

There is still no consensus regarding the relative benefits and risks of treating early stage patients with surgery, radiation therapy, hormonal therapy, or watchful waiting. Currently, and thankfully, about

80 percent of men diagnosed with prostate cancer have early stage disease.

To better understand the success rates, optimal timing, potential side effects and the long-term survival associated with these treatment options, in 1994 the National Cancer Institute launched the Prostate Cancer Outcomes Study (PCOS). By collecting comprehensive, long-term data on the health outcomes of various treatment options for prostate cancer, the PCOS will help patients, their families, and physicians make more informed decisions.

Some of the preliminary conclusions from the PCOS study have already been published. These include the following:

- Men with localized prostate cancer who are treated with radical prostatectomy are more likely to experience sexual and urinary dysfunction than those treated with external beam radiation therapy. Bowel dysfunction, on the other hand, is more common among men receiving external radiation therapy.

- Radical prostatectomy causes significant sexual dysfunction and some decline in urinary function.

- Imaging techniques such as bone scans, computerized tomography (CT), and magnetic resonance imaging (MRI) are showing that a small percentage of newly diagnosed prostate cancer cases have already metastasized (spread) beyond the prostate.

- Three factors were found to be the most accurate predictors of the spread of the cancer outside the prostate: Gleason score, PSA level, and stage of the disease.

Complementary and Alternative Therapies

Cancer patients are turning to so-called "complementary and alternative therapies" in extraordinary numbers. While some refer to such treatments as "complementary," and others as "alternative," and

TABLE III
Treatment Options for Prostate Cancer
Risks and Benefits

Treatment	Risks	Benefits	Comments
Surgery Radical Prostatectomy	Impotence; incontinence; infertility; frequency or urgency with urination.	Immediate removal of all cancer along with the prostate.	Long-term disability; need for catheter for several weeks; significant post-operative discomfort.
Radiation External Beam	Frequency, urgency or burning with urination; bloody urine; skin changes in area of radiation (including hair loss); bowel injury (diarrhea).	Destroys prostate cancer cells; decreases tumor size; decreases pain.	7-8 weeks of treatment, 5 days a week.
Brachytherapy	Bloody urine; impotence; frequency, urgency or burning with urination.	Minimally invasive; can be done as outpatient; minimizes change in lifestyle.	Until recently, considered experimental, but now many patients are excellent candidates for this treatment. May require a temporary urinary catheter.

TABLE III (continued)

Treatment Options for Prostate Cancer
Risks and Benefits

Treatment	Risks	Benefits	Comments
Hormonal Therapy	Impotence; infertility; decreased sexual drive; breast enlargement/pain; cardiovascular disease; nausea; vomiting; risk of osteoporosis with long-term use.	Relief from symptoms; decreases growth of prostate cancer; decreases size and viability of tumor (making it more amenable to other treatment options).	Not a cure. Simply slows growth of prostate cancer.
Chemotherapy	Nausea; vomiting; hair loss; mouth sores; anemia; fatigue.	Decreases pain; may slow cancer growth.	No proven beneficial effects of chemotherapy as adjuvant (additional) therapy as of this date. Not a cure.

still others as "complementary *and* alternative," there actually is a difference.

A therapy is generally called "complementary" when it is used *in addition to* conventional treatments. *Complementary* therapies are not intended to cure disease, but rather to help control symptoms and improve well-being. For example, a patient may practice meditation to reduce stress, or undergo acupuncture treatments to alleviate chronic pain. Other examples of complementary therapies include nutrition, taking vitamin supplements, massage, yoga, aromatherapy, biofeedback and guided imagery.

Alternative therapies refer to treatments that are intended to be used *instead of* conventional treatments. They are sometimes promoted as "cancer cures." Some alternative therapies, especially if taken in large doses, can counteract the benefits of standard medicines and skew test results. Examples of alternative therapies include mega-doses of vitamins or minerals, shark cartilage, and other such products. Many are expensive, some are harmful, and none have been proven effective. All are delaying important conventional medical treatment.

For prostate cancer, some of the more common complementary and alternative therapies include selenium, vitamin E, flaxseed, saw palmetto, soy, a Chinese herbal mixture called PC-SPES, and even aspirin. Encouragingly, a growing number of studies are also showing that a low fat diet and exercise are a great self-help option!

It is estimated that up to 75 percent of cancer patients are combining traditional medical treatments with complementary or alternative therapies. But *only a third* of them discuss their use of such therapies with their doctor.

Some doctors are concerned that the use of non-traditional treatments may lead patients to abandon standard medical care. However, it appears that many cancer patients view the use of complementary therapies as a way in which they can take control of their situation and become more personally involved in promoting a healthy recovery.

Understanding Your Treatment Options

Most complementary therapies, and many alternative therapies, are perfectly safe if used appropriately—and not at the expense of traditional medical treatment. You can only know for sure, however, if you talk with your doctor.

For example, PC SPES can have side effects similar to or worse than standard hormonal therapies (e.g., blood clots). Just because something is "herbal" doesn't mean it won't have side effects.

In addition, we can't caution you enough about treatments or therapies that promise you all, deliver nothing, and deplete your finances in the process! Don't allow yourself to get fooled. It could cost you more than money—it could cost you your health.

Clinical Trials

Most successful treatments used today began as clinical trials, which are studies designed to evaluate the safety and effectiveness of a new treatment. Those patients who participate in such trials are the first to potentially benefit from any improved therapies.

Clinical trials take place in many hospitals across the country and typically involve three *phases*:

Phase I – This is the first time that a new drug or treatment is tested in people. It usually involves only a small number of patients, but gives an early indication of a drug's or treatment's safety and potential effectiveness. Phase I studies are designed to find the safe and appropriate dose for testing in future studies. Side effects, while unpredictable, are carefully monitored.

Phase II – A phase II trial continues to test the safety of a drug or treatment, and attempts to measure how well it will actually work. A larger number of patients are enrolled in phase II trials so physicians can better assess the impact of the treatment. Side effects continue to be monitored.

Phase III – By this time, the new drug or treatment has shown early promise in treating a particular disease. The treatment will now be compared with a current standard. A participant will be randomly assigned to receive either the new treatment or a standard treatment (the "control group"). Phase III trials enroll large numbers of people and are conducted at medical centers nationwide.

All clinical trial participants receive the best care possible, and their reactions to all treatments are closely monitored. If the treatment does not seem to be helping, your doctor will remove you from the study. In addition, *you* may choose to leave the trial at any time. If you leave a clinical trial for any reason, standard care and treatment are still available as they were before. There is no penalty for leaving a trial.

Unfortunately, participation rates in clinical trials by eligible prostate cancer patients—especially older and minority patients—are extremely low. This has major implications for advances in prostate cancer treatment. Nearly all of the treatment options that are available to you today have come from previous prostate cancer clinical trials.

A common misunderstanding about contemporary clinical trials is the belief that you will receive no treatment if you are enrolled in the "control" group. Nothing could be further from the truth. In fact, if enrolled, you are guaranteed to receive, at the very least, the currently available treatment options. No "sugar pills!"

In addition, enrollment in clinical trials brings you "under the microscope." You may be observed, screened, tested and monitored far more carefully than someone who has chosen not to participate.

If you believe you are eligible for a clinical trial, or would simply like to know more about them, ask your doctor. You can also call the National Cancer Institute's Cancer Information Service at 1-800-4CANCER for more information.

Understanding Your Treatment Options

A Few Words About Pain

Not all cancer patients experience pain. Yet when pain does occur, it can often be treated effectively with nonprescription or prescription pain relievers. Even complementary approaches such as relaxation techniques and herbs can be used with good results.

Far too often, cancer pain is *not* adequately treated, and this can generate side effects of its own: headaches, weakness, sleeplessness, loss of appetite, anxiety, depression, and feelings of helplessness.

Sometimes pain is associated with your treatment, such as the discomfort following surgery or the skin irritation from radiation. This type of pain usually decreases over time, and medications are available to alleviate it during the course of treatment.

Pain can also be associated with the cancer itself. This can arise from a tumor causing pressure on adjacent organs, nerves, and tissues, or a cancer-related blockage of a particular blood vessel. When cancer metastasizes (spreads) to other organs, it can cause direct pain in those sites as well (i.e., the bones).

It is not always possible to identify or treat a single source of pain. In such cases, there are a number of pain-relief options. Medicines that relieve pain are called analgesics. Analgesics act on the nervous system to provide temporary relief from pain. Nonprescription pain relievers, sometimes called "over-the-counter" pain remedies, include aspirin, acetaminophen and ibuprofen.

For more severe pain, prescription pain relievers, in particular opioid narcotics, may be prescribed. These include: codeine, hydrocodone, hydromorphone, levorphanol, meperidine, methadone and morphine. Also, a transdermal (through the skin) fentanyl patch may be used for chronic pain management.

Sometimes pain can be relieved without non-prescription or prescription medicines. Such treatments include acupuncture, relaxation techniques, herbal supplements, and visualization/guided imagery.

Don't wait until you are experiencing significant pain to take your medication. Pain is much easier to control when it is mild rather than severe. You should take your pain medicine regularly and as often as your doctor recommends, or as often as you feel the need. While you may feel concerned about developing an addiction—forget it! You won't. **Be comfortable.** Don't hurt.

Treatment Follow-Up

At some point your treatment will end and RECOVERY will begin. Congratulations! An integral part of your long-term recovery process will be the appropriate follow-up appointments and tests to make sure that your treatment was successful and also, should your cancer return, to catch it in its earliest—and most treatable—stage.

While the post-treatment follow-up will differ from patient to patient, it is typical that you will see your doctor every 3 to 6 months in the first few years, getting regular PSA testing, digital rectal exams and a general medical evaluation. Be vigilant with your appointments. Medical follow-up is extremely important for both your initial recovery as well as your long-term health.

Understanding Your Treatment Options

My Notes

"Side Effects I'm Experiencing"
(And steps I can take to alleviate them!)

PART III:

Recovery

Recovery

Thanks to the many advances in prostate cancer treatment, especially in the past decade, more men are not only surviving prostate cancer, but are living healthy, disease-free lives long after treatment.

You are now a "prostate cancer survivor." **GREAT! You've recovered!** Finally your life will get back to normal.

However, as such, you will face a unique set of physical and emotional issues in the process. For example, regardless of age, the fear of recurrence will always (to some extent) be present. Don't let it take over your life!

Adequate nutrition and exercise will have a tremendous impact on your recovery—not to mention your overall health and well-being. Good nutrition is *absolutely essential*, but it is not always easy to maintain. For example, various treatments can suppress your appetite, as can anxiety and stress.

In general, if appetite becomes a concern, you may want to eat meals and snacks that include your favorite foods. Having more frequent, smaller meals may be helpful. Talk with your doctor or a nutritionist about a meal plan that meets your needs.

Exercise, even on a minimal scale, has been shown to have a profound impact on recovery in many cancer patients—not only in terms of physical recuperation but also for emotional well-being.

While your strength and stamina may vary at different times during your treatment and recovery, you may still be able to perform some type of moderate exercise. Remember, tailor it to your individual needs.

Emotional Issues

Let's step away from physical issues for a moment. The nagging fear of your cancer returning can have an *emotional* impact on your health.

Anxiety, sadness and temporary depression understandably accompany your diagnosis and treatment; these will subside with time. In the interim, there are medications available that can help, not to mention complementary therapies such as meditation and relaxation techniques.

Ongoing depression is a bit more serious and can have a profound bearing on your quality of life. It is therefore important to talk to your doctor if you suffer from extended bouts of anxiety, sadness, or significant changes in lifestyle that just aren't "you." Depression *can* be treated, but you must let your doctor know. Don't be embarrassed. **You are not alone.** In fact, your doctor may worry about you if you *don't* complain about feeling sad or depressed at some time following your diagnosis.

Don't conceal your feelings and concerns, especially from family, close friends and your healthcare team. There will be times during your treatment and recovery when everything might seem to be just too much to handle. That's normal, that's expected, and that's the time to reach for help. Don't deal with such feelings alone.

Fatigue and exhaustion can also have a direct impact on your emotional well-being. If you are refreshed and alert, you can handle more. So get plenty of rest, pace yourself, and make time for all of the activities that you enjoy!

Intimacy and Sexuality

Sexuality fulfills a significant need for closeness, and there is no reason that it cannot continue during your treatment and recovery. Yet some pervasive myths regarding sexuality and cancer still abound. Sex will *not* make your cancer worse and it *won't* cause a recurrence. In fact, the intimacy from sexual activity actually provides important emotional benefits throughout your recovery process. Your cancer will not be transmitted to your partner.

Sexual activity is usually safe during treatment. There may be times when sex may be temporarily painful, or when a period of rest and recuperation from *all* activities may be called for. But in general, if you're in the mood, enjoy it!

Prostate cancer, almost regardless of the treatment option you select, may result in some erectile dysfunction. However, a number of effective treatments are available to help you deal with this problem. These include medications, surgical procedures and externally assisted devices. (See Appendix VI.) All may result in an effective erection that will satisfy yourself and your partner. That's important for both of you. But keep in mind that even without an erection there are many ways to enjoy intimacy.

Be open and honest with your partner; hopefully your partner will be open and honest with you as well. Periods of time may pass where your desire for intimacy is subdued, followed by periods involving an intense need for intimacy. A little patience, a lot of communication, and an abundance of love can be especially important at this time in your life.

Financial Issues

Beyond its physical and emotional tolls, cancer can be a difficult financial challenge as well. You may have been working full-time when you were diagnosed and may need to take an extended leave of absence. In addition, your spouse and other family members may have to take time off from their work to be with you for support, comfort and that extra little need for attention.

Studies have shown that families can spend a significant proportion of their income on cancer care. It may be necessary to take out a loan or a second mortgage, spend savings, or get a second job to finance the needed treatments. Clearly this adds an additional stress to an already difficult situation.

Don't be embarrassed about any financial difficulties you might be having. Everyone—including most creditors—will understand. (This is *cancer*, not an overextended credit card.) Ask your doctor to refer you to a social worker who can recommend financial assistance programs. You may also be able to obtain assistance directly from your hospital, or from community organizations such as your church. *Ask!*

Consider talking to a financial advisor. A good one can negotiate extended payment plans, help you prioritize expenses, and perhaps suggest more effective ways to use your assets. You may also want to consider a program offered by the American Cancer Society called "Taking Charge of Money Matters," which includes workshops on many financial issues facing families with cancer. You can call them at 1-800-227-2345 for more information.

Cancer and Your Career

If you were working before your cancer diagnosis, count on returning to your job. You may appreciate it all the more!

When you return to work, you may find that some people simply aren't sure how to react. They may be scared, worried, or just don't understand what you are dealing with. Unfortunately, outdated notions still persist about cancer, especially if the disease has not touched someone personally.

In the beginning, you may have to take some time to simply talk with your co-workers about your illness and recovery. If you need help, ask your manager or someone in the Human Resources Department for assistance. If you work for a large company, there will likely be other employees who are cancer survivors. Consider forming a workplace cancer support group to discuss cancer- and job-related issues.

More than 80 percent of people with cancer return to work after their diagnosis. Yet 1 in 4 cancer survivors will experience some form of employment discrimination. If you feel that you are being treated unfairly, don't hesitate to take additional action.

Changing Jobs

If you are looking for a new job after your cancer treatment, it is important to anticipate that your cancer history may become an issue. Keep in mind that you have just overcome one of the biggest challenges in your life that you could possibly face. Take that **confidence** into the job interview! Additional suggestions from the National Cancer Institute include:

- Don't discriminate against yourself. Look at your current skills and capabilities and apply for jobs you know you can do, and do very well—perhaps better than anyone else.

- Organize your resume to your best advantage. For example, a chronological resume should avoid questions raised by your treatment or recovery. Avoid gaps, possibly by organizing your resume by skills or achievements instead of by dates of employment.

- Get a letter from your doctor (on office or hospital stationery) that explains your health situation to potential employers. Have your doctor specifically address your physical ability to perform the type of work you are seeking and to confirm that you are now in good health.

- Be honest about your cancer history if an employer or an application asks.

- Qualify your "yes" with **positive** statements about your current health.

- Avoid sounding defensive. Be confident!

- Don't volunteer health information if not asked. You have no legal responsibility to mention your cancer unless it directly relates to the job you seek. Information needs to be divulged on a "need-to-know" basis.

In addition, remember that anyone who asks about your personal medical history must present a written request, signed by you, to your doctor so that he/she may release any medical information, whether it involves cancer or any other condition.

Personal Support

You may be fortunate enough to have family members and close personal friends help you during treatment and recovery. Your cancer is affecting *them* as well—physically through fatigue from caregiving responsibilities, and emotionally with their understandable anxiety about your illness. Whatever emotions you are experiencing, chances are they are feeling many of the same.

Cancer causes great upheavals in the way family members interact, with traditional roles sometimes turned upside down and inside out. Parents might look to their children for emotional support at a time when the children themselves need it most. Teenagers might have to assume major household responsibilities. Young children can revert to infantile behavior as a way of dealing with their frustrations.

Patience, understanding, and examining what's truly important can often help families get through these times—they can become much stronger and closer as a result. Relax housekeeping standards, or have everyone pitch in to prepare meals. (It can be a lot of fun!) Children can, and often do, take on more household chores than they have handled before.

You will also develop an ongoing need for support from your healthcare team. This includes having a *two-way* dialogue with your doctor about any concerns that you may have. As mentioned before, take full advantage of your doctor's time during office visits:

- When going to meet your doctor or nurse, bring someone with you. It helps to have another person listen to and understand what is being said and to think of questions to ask during your consultation.

- Write out your questions beforehand; don't forget to discuss any issues.

- Write down or record the answers you get, and make sure you understand what you are hearing.

- Ask questions! If you feel that you are not receiving adequate answers to your concerns, ask where you can find them.

Support Groups

Is a support group for you? Cancer support groups are designed to provide a confidential atmosphere where you can talk frankly about the challenges that you are facing with others in a similar situation. Participants gather to exchange information, discuss practical problems (such as managing side effects), or simply to lend emotional support.

Your healthcare staff should be able to provide you with specific information about local support groups. Some meet informally with just survivors; others are directed by healthcare professionals. Take the time to find a support group that makes you feel comfortable and fits your specific needs. If you don't feel you want to be part of a support group, that's perfectly all right too.

Many prostate cancer survivors are surprised at how important their support group meetings become. There's nothing quite like sharing a concern or experience with someone who knows—on the most personal of levels—exactly what you're going through.

Coping With Recurrence

The news that the cancer has come back—recurred—is a time for understandable anxiety and fear. But it should *not* be a time for panic.

New advances in surgical techniques, radiation, chemotherapy and other treatments are becoming available on a consistent basis. On the immediate horizon are potentially *revolutionary* advances in cancer treatment, especially with our rapidly unfolding knowledge about the human genetic code.

At a time such as this, don't be afraid to show your emotions. Shock, grief and despair are normal—and understandable. Gather your family and friends around you. They have been invaluable since you were first diagnosed, and they will most certainly be supportive now.

Reassess your healthcare team if you feel the need. Make sure you are comfortable with your doctor and staff. Are they compassionate? Are they willing to consider a broad range of new treatment options? Are you satisfied with the care that you have received to date? If not, don't hesitate to get a second opinion, especially if you are considering new treatment options.

Most important of all—*don't give up!* Consider this as another bump in the road, although a rather difficult one. There are many, many men living well and disease-free today who have had recurrences of their own a long time ago. There is no reason why you can't be one of them!

Living With Advanced Disease

If your disease should become advanced, simple day-to-day activities that you once enjoyed may at times be more difficult, occasionally even overwhelming. There will be good days and bad days.

Keep in mind that the reality of advanced disease must *always* be balanced with the **hope** that one of the remarkable new treatments now emerging from clinical trials will be the perfect treatment developed just for *you*. Never, never give up hope.

In terms of your loved ones, however, be responsible. Update your will, prepare a Durable Power of Attorney for Health Care, and attend to any other matters of personal importance. Quite frankly, these are things that all of us should address long before *any* illness becomes an issue.

Some people find the diagnosis of cancer is a spur to do the fun, adventurous things they've always wanted to do but simply have put off. Go for it! Pursue travel plans, take on hobbies that have always interested you, or simply take the time to "catch your breath." Cancer and its treatment can be intensive, frustrating, exhausting, and often overwhelming. Step back and enjoy what truly makes you happy. Live life to the fullest!

APPENDICES

Appendix I:

Stages of Prostate Cancer

PROSTATE CANCER
Stage I

T1 Clinically inapparent tumor not palpable nor visible by imaging

T1a No M0 G1

T1a Tumor incidental histologic finding in 5% or less of tissue resected

G1 Well differentiated (slight anaplasia)

N0 No regional lymph node metastasis

M0 No distant metastasis

Used with the permission of the American Joint Committee on Cancer (AJCC®) Chicago, Illinois. The original source for this material is the AJCC® Cancer Staging Manual, 5th edition (1997) published by Lippincott-Raven Publishers, Philadelphia, Pennsylvania.

PROSTATE CANCER
Stage II

T1a N0 M0 G2, 3-4
T1b N0 M0 Any G

T1a Tumor incidental histologic finding in 5% or less of tissue resected

T1b Tumor incidental histologic finding in more than 5% of tissue resected

T1 clinically inapparent tumor not palpable nor visible by imaging

T1c N0 M0 Any G

T1c Tumor identified by needle biopsy (e.g., because of elevated PSA)

N0 No regional lymph node metastasis
M0 No distant metastasis

Used with the permission of the American Joint Committee on Cancer (AJCC®), Chicago, Illinois. The original source for this material is the AJCC® Cancer Staging Manual, 5th edition (1997) published by Lippincott-Raven Publishers, Philadelphia, Pennsylvania.

PROSTATE CANCER
Stage II (cont d)

T2 Tumor confined within prostate*

T2c N0 M0 Any G

T2a N0 M0 Any G
T2b N0 M0 Any G

T2a Tumor involves one lobe

T2b Tumor involves both lobes

N0 No regional lymph node metastasis

M0 No distant metastasis

*Note: Tumor found in one or both lobes by needle biopsy, but not palpable or reliably visible by imaging, classified as T1c.

Used with the permission of the American Joint Committee on Cancer (AJCC®) Chicago, Illinois. The original source for this material is the AJCC® Cancer Staging Manual, 5th edition (1997) published by Lippincott-Raven Publishers, Philadelphia, Pennsylvania.

PROSTATE CANCER
Stage III

T3 Tumor extends through the prostate capsule*

T3c N0 M0 Any G

T3a N0 M0 Any G
T3b N0 M0 Any G

T3a Extracapsular extension (unilateral or bilateral)

T3b Tumor invades seminal vesicle(s)

N0 No regional lymph node metastasis

M0 No distant metastasis

*Note: Invasion into the prostatic apex or into (but not beyond) the prostatic capsule is not classified as T3, but as T2.

Used with the permission of the American Joint Committee on Cancer (AJCC®) Chicago, Illinois. The original source for this material is the AJCC® Cancer Staging Manual, 5th edition (1997) published by Lippincott-Raven Publishers, Philadelphia, Pennsylvania.

PROSTATE CANCER
Stage IV

T4 Tumor is fixed or invades adjacent structures other than seminal vesicles: bladder neck, external sphincter, rectum, levator muscles, and/or pelvic wall

T4 N0 M0 Any G

Any T N1 M0 Any G
Any T Any N M1 Any G

N1 Metastasis in regional lymph node or nodes

M1   Distant metastases
M1a Nonregional lymph node(s)
M1b Bone(s)
M1c Other site(s)

Used with the permission of the American Joint Committee on Cancer (AJCC®) Chicago, Illinois. The original source for this material is the AJCC® Cancer Staging Manual, 5th edition (1997) published by Lippincott-Raven Publishers. Philadelphia. Pennsylvania.

Appendix II:

Prostate Cancer Treatment Options

Prostate Cancer Treatment Options

According to currently acceptable guidelines, prostate cancer patients are generally placed into one of the following categories:

1. Low Risk
2. Intermediate Risk
3. High Risk
4. Very High Risk

Because prostate cancer, fortunately, tends to be a slow-growing cancer, "watchful waiting" may be an appropriate treatment strategy at any risk level.

Watchful Waiting

We do not like the term "watchful waiting" because it implies something bad will happen. Rather, the term should be interpreted in a positive context: it appears that nothing bad will happen to you from having prostate cancer.

Watchful waiting does not mean "do nothing." It implies monitoring until something changes; realizing it may not, but also that treatment may be necessary if changes occur.

Watchful waiting may be appropriate as a treatment strategy if at least one of the following criteria are met:

- Less than 10 year survival is anticipated due to older age or other underlying diseases.

- Gleason Score - 2 to 4, and a stable PSA with a rigorous monitoring schedule.

Treatment Recommendations:

- Do nothing at this time.
- Careful monitoring that would include at least an annual digital rectal exam (DRE) and PSA test.

Notes:

Patients in this category may have Stage I or Stage A cancer. Alternatively, it may be classified as Stage T1. This means that the cancer cannot be felt during a digital rectal exam. It may have been found incidentally when surgery was done for another reason, usually for benign prostatic hyperplasia (BPH). There is no evidence that the cancer has spread outside the prostate.

A small nodule (Stage B1) may be appropriate for watchful waiting if other criteria are met.

Low Risk

Low risk means that the cancer was caught in an early stage of the disease (T1 or T2) and probably has not spread beyond the prostate gland. Patients are called "low risk" because they have a low risk of cancer having spread beyond the prostate gland, and a low risk of dying of prostate cancer if they are treated with surgery or radiation. To be classified as low risk, the following criteria must be met:

- Stage T1a - T2a:
  – T1a – A tumor was found incidentally in tissue that was resected (removed) for other reasons; it involves less than 5 percent of the tissue removed.
  – T1b – A tumor was found incidentally in tissue resected (removed) for other reasons; it involves *more* than 5 percent of the tissue removed.

Prostate Cancer Treatment Options

- T1c – A tumor was found based solely on PSA screening.
- T2a – A palpable tumor (it can be felt) involving only one side of the prostate (left or right).
- PSA - 10 ng/ml or less.
- Gleason Score – 2 to 6.

Recommendations:

- Radiation therapy (external beam or brachytherapy).
- Radical prostatectomy.
- Watchful waiting.

Notes:

A Stage II or Stage B cancer may be classified as low risk. The tumor can be felt during a digital rectal exam. However, there is no evidence that the cancer has spread outside the prostate. Prostate cancer tumors in the low risk category can also be classified as T1 or T2 as follows:

- T1 – The tumor cannot be felt during a digital rectal exam, but cancer cells are found in a prostate biopsy or prostatectomy specimen. T1 cancers can be subdivided as: *T1a* (less than 5 percent of the removed tissue is cancerous); *T1b* (more than 5 percent of the removed tissue is cancerous); *T1c* (a tumor was found based solely on PSA screening).
- T2 – The tumor can be felt during a digital rectal exam, but the cancer appears to be confined to the prostate gland. T2 cancers can be subdivided as: *T2a* (the tumor involves only one side of the prostate); or *T2b* (the tumor involves both sides of the prostate).

Intermediate Risk

Prostate cancer patients who are considered to be at intermediate risk have cancer that probably has not spread beyond the prostate. Men in this group may benefit from more aggressive treatment (radical prostatectomy or radiation), especially if they have a longer life expectancy. These patients otherwise have "low risk" disease, but one of the following adverse features is present:

- T2b – Palpable tumor (it can be felt) involving more than half of one lobe, but not both lobes.
- PSA – 10 ng/ml or higher, but less than 20 ng/ml.
- Gleason Score – 7.

Recommendations:

- Radiation therapy (external beam or brachytherapy).
- Radical prostatectomy.
- Hormone ablation to shrink tumor size may be indicated prior to radiation or radical prostatectomy.

Notes:

T2a tumors may be classified as low risk if other criteria are met. T2b lesions are generally intermediate risk or higher.

High Risk

If the cancer has spread to both sides of the prostate and beyond, it may be considered as high risk. If so, radical prostatectomy, radiation and hormonal therapy may all be appropriate treatment options. To be classified as high risk, at least *two* of the following adverse criteria must be met:

- T2b – Palpable tumor (it can be felt); both right and left sides of the prostate are involved.
- PSA – Greater than 10 ng/ml.
- Gleason Score – 7.

Or any single criteria of:
- T3 – Palpable tumor beyond the prostate.
- PSA > 20.
- Gleason Score ≥ 8.

Prostate Cancer Treatment Options

Recommendations:

- Radical prostatectomy or external beam radiation with or without pre-operative hormonal therapy.
- Combined external beam and implant radiation.

Notes:

A Stage III or Stage C cancer is classified as high risk. The cancer has spread locally outside the prostate to nearby tissues. However, there is no evidence of distant (metastatic) disease.

Very High Risk

Very high risk patients are those at high risk for metastatic disease (cancer that has spread beyond the prostate) but with no evidence of metastatic disease at present. At least *two* of the following criteria must be present for the cancer to be considered very high risk:

- T3 – The cancer has spread to the connective tissue next to the prostate or to the seminal vesicles, but does not involve any other organs. T3 cancers can be divided as: *T3a* (the cancer has spread outside the prostate but not to the seminal vesicles); or *T3b* (the cancer has spread to involve the seminal vesicles).
- PSA > 20 ng/ml.
- Gleason Score – 8 to 10.

Recommendations:

- External beam radiation with long-term hormonal ablation therapy.
- Possible radical prostatectomy.
- Possible combination therapy with external beam radiation and brachytherapy.

"I Flunked My PSA!"

Notes:

A Stage IV or Stage D cancer has spread beyond the confines of the prostate to lymph nodes, bones or to other parts of the body. Local therapy alone will be insufficient. Additional treatments are necessary.

My Notes

"My Current Treatment Strategy"
(And new treatments I might consider!)

Appendix III:

Common Prostate Cancer Drugs: Hormonal Agents

Appendix III

Common Prostate Cancer Drugs: Hormonal Agents

Drug (Trade Name) Manufacturer	Indications	Possible Side Effects	Method of Administration
LH-RH* AGONISTS			
Leuprolide (Lupron®) Tap Pharmaceuticals	For the treatment of prostate cancer.	Hot flashes, depression, edema, headache, weight gain, breast tenderness, impotence.	Intramuscular injection; Depot (sustained release injection)
Goserelin (Zolodex®) AstraZeneca Pharmaceuticals	For the treatment of prostate cancer.	Hot flashes, depression, edema, headache, weight gain, breast tenderness, impotence.	Subcutaneous pellet injection (sustained release injection)

* LH-RH - Luteinizing Hormone-Releasing Hormone

Common Prostate Cancer Drugs

Drug (Trade Name) Manufacturer	Indications	Possible Side Effects	Method of Administration
ANTI-ANDROGENS			
Bicalutamide (Casodex®) AstraZeneca Pharmaceuticals	For the treatment of prostate cancer.	Hot flashes, liver dysfunction, diarrhea, fatigue, breast enlargement/tenderness.	Oral (tablet)
Flutamide (Eulexin®) Schering Oncology	For the treatment of prostate cancer.	Hot flashes, liver dysfunction, diarrhea, nausea, breast enlargement/tenderness.	Oral (tablet)
Nilutamide (Nilandron®) Hoechst Marion Roussel	For the treatment of prostate cancer.	Hot flashes, liver dysfunction, diarrhea, fatigue, decreased night vision.	Oral (tablet)
Megestrol Acetate (Megace®) Bristol-Myers Squibb	For the treatment of prostate cancer.	Hot flashes, tumor pain, edema, increased appetite.	Oral (tablet)
Ketoconazole (Nizoral®) Janssen	For the treatment of prostate cancer.	Breast tenderness, sugar intolerance, muscle pain.	Oral (tablet)
Estrogens	For the treatment of prostate cancer.	Blood clots, breast tenderness, decreased libido.	Oral (tablet)

Appendix IV:

Common Prostate Cancer Drugs: Chemotherapy Agents

Appendix IV

Common Prostate Cancer Drugs: Chemotherapy Agents

Drug (Trade Name) Manufacturer	Indications	Possible Side Effects	Method of Administration
Docetaxel (Taxotere®) Aventis	For the treatment of hormone refractory prostate cancer	Hair loss, bone marrow suppression, hypersensitivity, edema, nail changes.	Injection (IV)
Epoitin Alfa (Procrit®) Ortho-Biotech	For the treatment of anemia associated with chemotherapy or radiation.	Headaches, joint and bone pain, nausea.	Injection (IV), or subcutaneous injection
Estramustine Phosphate (EMCYT®) Aventis	For the treatment of hormone refractory prostate cancer.	Fatigue, nausea, vomiting, edema, blood clots, bone marrow suppression.	Injection (IV); Oral dosage may be available soon.
Etoposide (VePesid®) Bristol-Myers Squibb	For the treatment of hormone refractory prostate cancer.	Hair loss, bone marrow suppression, low blood pressure.	Injection (IV)

Common Prostate Cancer Drugs

Drug (Trade Name) Manufacturer	Indications	Possible Side Effects	Method of Administration
Mitoxantrone (Novantrone®) Immunex	For the treatment of hormone refractory prostate cancer.	Hair loss, bone marrow suppression, heart damage.	Injection (IV)
Paclitaxel (Taxol®) Bristol-Myers Squibb	For the treatment of hormone refractory prostate cancer.	Hair loss, bone marrow suppression, neuropathy, hypersensitivity.	Injection (IV)
Vinblastine (Velban®) Eli Lilly	For the treatment of hormone refractory prostate cancer.	Hair loss, bone marrow suppression, neuropathy, vein irritation.	Injection (IV)

* Side effects listed in these Appendices are not all-inclusive. Nearly all cancer drugs cause suppression of blood counts (anemia), resulting in an increased susceptibility to infections and fatigue. It is important to report any symptoms to your healthcare team.

Appendix V:

Common Anti-Nausea Medications

Appendix V

Common Anti-Nausea Medications

Drug (Trade Name) Manufacturer	Indications	Possible Side Effects	Method of Administration
Dolasetron (Anzemet®) Aventis Pharmaceuticals	Prevent/treat nausea and vomiting following chemotherapy/surgery.	Irregular heartbeat, diarrhea, abdominal pain, headache.	Oral (tablet) Injection (IV)
Granisetron (Kytril®) Glaxo SmithKline	Prevent/treat nausea and vomiting following chemotherapy/surgery.	Headaches, constipation, anemia.	Oral (tablet) Injection (IV)
Ondansetron (Zofran®) Glaxo SmithKline	Prevent/treat nausea and vomiting following chemotherapy/surgery.	Headaches, fatigue, diarrhea, constipation, muscle pain.	Oral (tablet) Injection (IV)
Dexamethasone (generic)	To prevent delayed-onset nausea and vomiting from chemotherapy.	Irregular heartbeat, euphoria, insomnia, abdominal pain, hyperglycemia, irritability, edema.	Oral (suspension and tablet), Injection (IV)
Metoclopramide (generic)	To treat breakthrough and delayed nausea and vomiting that may occur from chemotherapy.	Restlessness, seizures, abdominal pain, diarrhea, sedation.	Oral (suspension and tablet), Injection (IV)

Common Prostate Cancer Drugs

Drug (Trade Name) Manufacturer	Indications	Possible Side Effects	Method of Administration
Prochlorperazine (Compazine®) Smithkline Beecham	Prevent/treat nausea and vomiting following chemotherapy/surgery.	Sedation, dry mouth, restlessness.	Oral (tablet and suspension), Injection (IV)

Appendix VI:

Prostate Cancer and Sexuality

Prostate Cancer and Sexuality

Nearly 70 percent of men who have been treated for prostate cancer experience some level of sexual dysfunction, primarily difficulties with erection and a decrease in sexual desire.

The physical side effects from cancer and its treatment are often cited as the obvious reasons for these sexual difficulties, but psychological and emotional factors are sometimes just as debilitating.

Psychological factors that may impact sexuality include depression, confusion, anxiety, guilt, stress caused by the diagnosis of cancer, and changes in "body image" following surgery and adjuvant (additional) therapies.

The degree to which the resulting sexual dysfunction impacts a person's quality of life varies dramatically from patient to patient. Keep in mind that medicines as well as other treatment options can often minimize this impact, if not eliminate it altogether.

In the past few years, many of the sexual side effects of cancer treatment have been researched with fervor. And yet, a surprising number of doctors still don't discuss sexual difficulties with their patients, let alone recognize the symptoms that may be leading up to such difficulties.

Depression and Sexual Desire

Depression is often the major underlying factor for patients experiencing a loss of sexual desire or the inability to enjoy sexual pleasure. Depression can have other far-reaching consequences as well. It is therefore important to talk with your doctor if you feel you are experiencing any symptoms of depression.

Often depression is temporary and accompanies the understandable emotional trauma of a diagnosis of cancer and its treatment. Staying active is a good way to fight depression and reduce stress. Exercise has also been shown to be an excellent technique to make you feel better about yourself. In addition, there are a number of relaxation techniques that may help you cope at various times during your treatment and recovery.

What doctors call "clinical depression" has a number of symptoms, including the lack of interest in sex, a lack of interest in things that usually give you pleasure, and even being unable to feel pleasure at all. Often these feelings are associated with insomnia, changes in eating habits, fatigue, difficulty concentrating, and feelings of worthlessness and hopelessness.

Depression can often be treated with medications to improve your sleep, enhance your appetite, increase your energy and, in general, improve your ability to feel pleasure. In turn, your self-esteem and desire for sexual activity will thrive. But you must ask your doctor. It is nothing to be ashamed of, and it could dramatically change your life for the better.

Myths Surrounding Sexuality and Cancer

Sexuality is just one aspect of our need for closeness, but it is a very important one—especially during treatment and recovery. Even when sex becomes difficult, the physical expression of caring remains an integral part of the coping process.

Unfortunately, some pervasive myths regarding sexuality and cancer still abound; most are unfounded and many are based on simple misunderstandings of the disease and the treatments for it.

For example, cancer is *not* contagious. Cancer cannot be passed from one person to another through sexual contact—or in any other way for that matter. Cancer is not contagious regardless of the type of sex involved, including everything from touching and kissing to intercourse and oral sex.

A cancer cell simply cannot leave one person and begin growing in another. Not only are cancer cells—and all cells—fragile, but another person's immune system will immediately recognize a foreign cell that is not "one of its own" and destroy it.

Also, sex will not make cancer worse or more likely to spread. Whether the cancer spreads or goes into remission is completely independent of sexual activity. In fact, the intimacy derived from sex may actually provide important emotional support and benefits. Who knows, the hormonal and chemical changes that take place in the body during orgasm may even have some palliative effects.

During treatment and recovery from cancer, sexual activity is usually safe. However, there may be times when it is temporarily painful, or when a period of rest and recuperation from *all* activities is called for. Such times may include the period immediately following surgery. In any case, check with your doctor.

Radiation treatments to certain areas may make your skin more tender or susceptible to breakdown and perhaps infection. Different positions during sex, or different ways of achieving orgasm that do not involve the treated area, may be helpful.

At times during treatment your immune system may be weakened, especially during chemotherapy or radiation therapy. You may be more susceptible to infections, including sexually transmitted diseases. Simple precautions, such as using a condom, should be considered.

While undergoing external beam radiation therapy, sex will not expose your partner to radiation. In fact, radiation exposure is minimal for you as the patient, and even then it is specifically targeted at the cancer itself. External radiation therapy has the immediate impact of destroying cancer cells but it does not linger in the body. Therefore, it does not expose your partner to any radiation risk.

In the case of radioactive seed implants (brachytherapy) for the treatment of prostate cancer, some special precautions may need to be taken. While there is no long-term risk of radiation exposure to yourself or others, you will be asked to use a condom during the first few months after the procedure to be absolutely safe. You should also avoid close and prolonged contact with pregnant women and newborn infants for a few months.

There are no risks to your partner from the chemotherapy drugs you may be taking, although during treatment a very low level of such drugs and their breakdown products may be present in the semen. Ask your doctor if this applies to the drugs you are taking. If so, it may be appropriate to use condoms around the time you are receiving your chemotherapy.

Finally, some outdated and unfounded religious fears about cancer may stem from the image that both sex and cancer are "unclean," or that the disease may be a "punishment for past sins." Some people even promise to give up sex as a sacrifice in return for a cancer cure. Few religions support such a harsh view of either cancer or sexuality. Discuss such concerns with your priest, minister, rabbi, imam, or other religious leader.

Communication is Crucial

If you are wondering whether sexual activity would cause a problem during treatment, ask your doctor. The answer may vary at different times and for different people. But common sense, and a simple question to your doctor, may be all that is necessary.

Communication is just as important with your partner, if not more so. Sexual desire may fluctuate during treatment. Long periods of time may pass where your desire for intimacy is subdued, followed by periods involving an intense need for closeness. Beyond the physical impact of the disease, anxiety, fears, and even depression can impact intimacy.

When it comes to sexuality and cancer, many fears unfortunately still abound. Most of them are unfounded—but *all* of them should be communicated.

Physical Side Effects of Treatment Options

Certain procedures to treat cancer can affect male sexual function. For example, some procedures may damage the nerves or blood vessels that are necessary for a male to achieve an unassisted erection. Even anxiety from the cancer itself can cause a loss of desire and difficulty in achieving erection.

Often these problems are temporary, although it may take months or even years for sexual performance to return to normal for some men. Other treatments, however, can have a permanent (although not necessarily debilitating), impact on sexual function.

Just as with any cancer treatment, some patients fare better than others in terms of side effects. Younger patients often do better than older patients, but there is no discernible pattern as to who will recover sexual function and who will not.

Most prostate cancer treatments will have some affect on male sexuality.

Radical Prostatectomy

A radical prostatectomy is used to treat locally confined prostate cancer and involves the surgical removal of the prostate gland, the seminal vesicles and pelvic nodes.

The introduction of nerve-sparing techniques for radical prostatectomy in 1982 and subsequent refinements to the procedure in recent years have enabled the preservation of sexual functioning in many more patients. For some men with more extensive disease, however, nerve sparing surgery is not possible.

The success rates in preserving erections with nerve-sparing techniques differ from center to center. In experienced centers, 70 to 80 percent of patients under age 60 with normal preoperative erections will recover sexual function. The numbers fall with increasing age; about 60 percent of those in their 60s, and 40 to 50 percent of those over 70, eventually recover erectile function. Erections usually return three to six months postoperatively and improve for the following two years.

Clinical trials aimed at reducing the size of the tumor before surgery may result in decreased surgical side effects. Such approaches include preoperative chemotherapy, hormonal therapy or radiation. In addition, due to the prostate specific antigen (PSA) blood screening test, smaller cancers are being detected. Early detection may translate into less extensive surgery with fewer complications.

Orchiectomy and Hormonal Treatments

An orchiectomy is the removal of one (unilateral) or both (bilateral) testicles, but not the scrotum. It is used to treat prostate and testicular cancer. Surgery to remove the testicle through an incision in the groin is called a radical inguinal orchiectomy.

Although a surgical procedure, bilateral orchiectomy is actually a hormonal intervention. Testosterone levels fall and sexual function is affected in 80 percent of these patients. Problems with desire, arousal and orgasm can occur.

Complete androgen blockade, and the administration of other medications or anti-androgens, can result in erectile difficulties. Additional side effects may include fatigue, mood swings, depression and hot flashes. Osteoporosis (weakening of the bones) may also occur with prolonged therapy. Different treatments are available to alleviate most of the above symptoms.

If a bilateral orchiectomy is performed, artificial testicles, called prostheses, can be placed in the scrotum. The implants have the weight and feel of a normal testicle but do not have the ability to function like one. They are for cosmetic purposes only.

Radiation Treatment

The higher the total dose of radiation and the wider the area that is irradiated, the greater the chance that a problem with erection will develop. Both external beam radiation and seed implant radiation (brachytherapy) can damage the nerves and arteries that carry blood to the penis. As the irradiated zone heals, the walls of the arteries can become scarred, losing their elasticity and resulting in decreased blood flow to the penis.

It is estimated that 40 to 60 percent of men who receive radiation treatment will develop some problem with erection. This change develops most often after the first year or so following radiotherapy. Some men continue to have full erections but lose them before reaching climax. Others no longer get firm erections at all.

After radiation to the prostate, some men ejaculate only a few drops of semen. In addition, toward the end of the radiation treatment, some men may feel a sharp pain as they ejaculate. The pain results from irritation within the urethra (the urinary tube through the penis). It should decrease within several months after the end of treatment.

In a small percentage of men, testosterone production may slow after pelvic radiation. The testicles are affected either by a mild dose of scattered radiation or even by the general stress of cancer treatment. However, testosterone levels usually recover within six months after radiation therapy.

Treatment Options for Erectile Dysfunction

Many of the sexual side effects from prostate cancer treatment are temporary. But for those that are not, there are a growing number of medical and surgical interventions that may help restore some or all of your sexual function. These include various medications, surgical procedures and externally assisted devices.

All may result in an effective erection that will satisfy you and your partner. That's important for both of you. Besides satisfaction, it is therapy—you are still an intimate couple!

There are three broad treatment options for erectile dysfunction: medications (including Viagra®, Yohimbine, vasodilator therapy, and injections); surgery (implants); and externally assisted devices.

The oral medications currently available have a broad range of effectiveness. Among the most promising is sildenfil (Viagra®), which acts by promoting relaxation of the blood vessels in the penis so that more blood rushes into the penis, causing an erection. In order for sildenfil to work, you must have at least one viable nerve bundle.

Specifically, sildenfil relaxes the blood vessels by delaying the action of enzymes called phosphodiesterases in the penis. Sildenfil helps to maintain an erection when the penis is physically stimulated, such as during intercourse. Without this physical stimulation, sildenfil will not work effectively.

For men with mild erection difficulties, Yohimbine, a derivative of the bark of an African tree, may be an option. Side effects include anxiety, nervousness or a rapid heartbeat. These can sometimes be avoided by starting with low doses and working up to the usual three-times daily dosage.

Vasodilator injections (such as Caverject®) act in the same way as sildenfil by causing relaxation of the blood vessels in the penis so that more blood flows into the penis, resulting in an erection. They can be injected directly into the penile tissues. Erections are usually pro-

Prostate Cancer and Sexuality

duced in 10 to 15 minutes and last between 15 and 45 minutes. Side effects may include bruising at the site of the injection, aching of the penis, scarring and prolonged erections.

Surgical implants can be placed inside the penis, although this invasive procedure is often used as a last resort because it may preclude other treatment alternatives. Some implants keep the penis in an erect position; others can be inflated to achieve an erection as needed. Side effects include infection, an improper fit, nerve damage to the penis, and injury to the urethra. In addition, the implants can occasionally become defective.

Vacuum-assisted devices are comprised of cylinders that are placed on the outside of the penis. They are attached to a hand-held pump that creates a vacuum to pull blood into the penis, causing an erection. The erection is maintained by placing a rubber band at the base of the penis and it may last for up to 30 minutes.

Another technique involves the use of a vibrator on the underside of the penis to stimulate blood flow and erection. This can be used in concert with your partner, providing stimulation for both of you.

The advantage of these devices is that they are simple and non-invasive, although they are somewhat inconvenient to use.

Finally, if you are going to have cancer treatment that might lead to infertility, you may want to ask your doctor about sperm banking (freezing sperm before treatment so it can be used in the future). This procedure can allow some men to produce children after the loss of fertility.

Appendix VII:

Glossary of Prostate Cancer Terms

Glossary of Prostate Cancer Terms

A

Adrenal glands: A pair of small glands, one located on top of each kidney. They produce steroid hormones, adrenaline and noradrenaline, which help control heart rate, blood pressure, and small amounts of male hormones.

Aminoglutethimide: An anticancer drug used to decrease the production of sex hormones (estrogen or testosterone) and suppress the growth of tumors that need sex hormones to continue to grow.

Androgens: A family of hormones that promote the development and maintenance of male sex characteristics.

Antiandrogens: Drugs used to block the production or interfere with the action of male sex hormones.

B

Benign: Not cancerous; does not invade nearby tissue or spread to other parts of the body.

Benign prostatic hyperplasia: A noncancerous condition in which an overgrowth of prostate tissue pushes against the urethra and the bladder, possibly blocking the flow of urine. Also called benign prostatic hypertrophy or BPH.

Bicalutamide (Casodex®): An anticancer drug that belongs to the family of drugs called antiandrogens.

Biological therapy: Treatment to stimulate or restore the ability of the immune system to fight infection and disease. Also used to lessen side effects that may be caused by some cancer treatments. Also known as immunotherapy, biotherapy, or biological response modifier (BRM) therapy.

Biopsy: The removal of cells or tissues for examination under a microscope. When only a sample of tissue is removed, the procedure is called an incisional biopsy or core biopsy. When an entire tumor or lesion is removed, the procedure is called an excisional biopsy. When a sample of tissue or fluid is removed with a needle, the procedure is called a needle biopsy or fine-needle aspiration.

Bladder: The organ that stores urine.

Brachytherapy: A procedure in which radioactive material sealed in needles, seeds, wires, or catheters is placed directly into or near a tumor. Also called internal radiation, implant radiation, or interstitial radiation therapy.

C

Cancer: A term for diseases in which abnormal cells divide without control. Cancer cells can invade nearby tissues and can spread through the bloodstream and lymphatic system to other parts of the body.

Catheter: A thin, flexible tube through which fluids enter or leave the body, such as a tube to drain urine.

Chemotherapy: Treatment with anticancer drugs. Also known as systemic therapy.

Clinical trial: A research study that tests how well new medical treatments or other interventions work in people. Each study is designed to test new methods of screening, prevention, diagnosis, or treatment of a particular disease.

Complete androgen blockade: Therapy used to drastically reduce male sex hormones (androgens) in the body. This may be done with surgery (bilateral orchiectomy), hormones, or as a combination of these treatments. Also known as total androgen blockade.

Cryosurgery: Treatment performed with an instrument that freezes and destroys abnormal tissues.

Cystoscopy: Examination of the bladder and urethra using a thin, lighted instrument (cystoscope) inserted into the urethra. Tissue samples can be removed and examined under a microscope to determine whether a particular disease is present.

D

Digital rectal examination (DRE): An examination in which a doctor inserts a lubricated, gloved finger into the rectum to feel for any abnormalities of the prostate or rectum.

Dry orgasm: Sexual climax without the release of semen or other seminal fluids from the penis.

E

Ejaculation: The release of semen through the penis during orgasm.

External radiation: Radiation therapy that uses an x-ray machine to aim high-energy rays at a particular cancer. Also called external-beam radiation.

F

Finasteride (Proscar®): A drug used to reduce the amount of a major male hormone, DHT, produced by the body.

Flutamide (Eulexin®): An anticancer drug that belongs to the family of drugs called antiandrogens.

G

Gene: The functional and physical unit of heredity passed from parent to offspring. Genes are strands of DNA.

Genitourinary system: The parts of the body that play a major role in reproduction and getting rid of waste products in the form of urine.

Goserelin (Zolodex®): A drug that belongs to the family of drugs called gonadotropin-releasing hormone analogues. Goserelin is used to block hormone production in the ovaries or testicles.

Grade: The grade of a tumor depends on how abnormal the cancer cells look under a microscope and how quickly the tumor is likely to grow and spread. Grading systems differ for each type of cancer.

H

Hormonal therapy: Treatment of cancer by removing, blocking, or adding hormones. Also called endocrine therapy.
Hormones: Chemicals produced by glands in the body which control the actions of certain organs.

I

Impotent: Unable to have an unassisted erection during sex.

Incontinence: Inability to control the flow of urine from the bladder (urinary incontinence) or the escape of stool from the rectum (fecal incontinence).

Internal radiation: A procedure in which radioactive material, delivered by needles to implant seeds, wires, or catheters is placed directly into or near the tumor. Also called brachytherapy, implant radiation, or interstitial radiation therapy.

Intravenous pyelogram: A series of x-rays of the kidneys, ureters, and bladder. The dye is injected intravenously and concentrates in the urine, which outlines the kidneys, ureters, and bladder on the x-rays.

K

Ketoconazole (Nizoral®): A drug that treats an infection caused by a fungus. It is also used as a treatment for prostate cancer because it can block the production of the male sex hormone testosterone.

L

Leuprolide (Lupron®): A drug that belongs to a family of drugs called gonadotropin-releasing hormone analogues. It is used to block hormone production in the testicles.

Local therapy: Treatment that affects cells in the tumor directly and any area close to it.

Luteinizing hormone-releasing hormone agonist: LH-RH agonist. A drug that inhibits the secretion of sex hormones. In men, LH-RH agonist cause testosterone levels to fall.

Lymph node: A rounded mass of lymphatic tissue that is surrounded by a capsule of connective tissue. Also known as a lymph gland. Lymph nodes, connected by lymphatic vessels, are found throughout the body and are responsible for filtering the blood of infectious agents as well as cancer cells.

Lymphatic system: The tissues and organs that produce, store, and carry white blood cells that fight infection and other diseases. This system includes the bone marrow, spleen, thymus, lymph nodes and a network of thin tubes that carry lymph and white blood cells. These tubes branch, like blood vessels, into all the tissues of the body.

M

Malignant: Cancerous; a growth with a tendency to invade and destroy nearby tissues and spread to other parts of the body.

Medical oncologist: A doctor who specializes in diagnosing and treating cancer using chemotherapy, hormonal therapy, and biological therapy. A medical oncologist often serves as the main caretaker of someone who has cancer and coordinates any treatment protocols provided by other specialists.

Metastasis: The spread of cancer from one part of the body to another. Tumors formed from cells that have spread are called "secondary tumors" and contain cells that are like those in the original (primary) tumor.

P

Pathologist: A doctor who identifies diseases by studying cells and tissues under a microscope.

Glossary of Prostate Cancer Terms

Prostate gland: A gland in the male reproductive system just below the bladder. It surrounds a part of the urethra, the canal that empties the bladder, and produces a fluid that forms a major part of semen.

Prostate-specific antigen (PSA): A substance produced by the prostate gland that may be found in an increased amount in the blood of men who have prostate cancer, benign prostatic hyperplasia, and infection or inflammation of the prostate.

Prostatectomy: An operation to remove part or all of the prostate. Radical (or total) prostatectomy is the removal of the entire prostate gland and the lymph nodes around it.

Prostatic acid phosphatase (PAP): An enzyme produced by the prostate.

R

Radiation oncologist: A doctor who specializes in using radiation to treat cancer.

Radiation therapy: The use of high-energy radiation from x-rays, protons, gamma rays, neutrons, and other sources to kill cancer cells and shrink tumors. Radiation may come from a machine outside the body (external-beam radiation therapy), or it may come from radioactive material placed in the body in the area near cancer cells (internal radiation therapy, implant radiation, or brachytherapy).

Rectum: The last 6 inches of the large intestine.

Recur: To occur again. Recurrence is the return of a cancer, at the same site as the original (primary) tumor or in another location.

Risk factor: A habit, trait, condition, or genetic alteration that increases your chance of developing a disease.

S

Scrotum: In males, the external sac that contains the testicles.

Semen: The fluid that is released through the penis during orgasm. Semen is made up of sperm from the testicles and fluid from the prostate and other sex glands.

Seminal fluid: Fluid from the prostate and other sex glands that helps transport sperm out of the man's body during orgasm.

Sonogram: A computer picture of areas inside the body created by bouncing sound waves off organs and other tissues. Also called an ultrasonogram or ultrasound.

Staging: Performing exams and tests to learn the extent of a cancer within the body, especially whether the disease has spread from the original site to other parts of the body.

Systemic therapy: Treatment that uses substances that travel through the bloodstream, reaching and affecting cells all over the body. Also known as chemotherapy.

T

Testicles: The two egg-shaped glands found inside the scrotum. They produce sperm and male hormones. Also called testes.

Testosterone: A hormone that promotes the development and maintenance of male sexual characteristics.

Total androgen blockade: Therapy used to drastically reduce male sex hormones (androgens) in the body. This may be done with surgery (bilateral orchiectomy), hormones, or as a combination of these treatments. Also known as complete androgen blockade.

Transurethral resection of the prostate (TURP): Surgical procedure to remove tissue from the prostate using an instrument inserted through the urethra.

Tumor: An abnormal mass of tissue that results from excessive cell division. It may be benign (not cancerous) or malignant (cancerous).

U

Ultrasonography: A procedure in which sound waves (called ultrasound) are bounced off tissues and the echoes are converted to a picture (sonogram).

Urethra: The tube through which urine leaves the body. It empties urine from the bladder, and passes through the center of the prostate.

Urologist: A doctor who specializes in diseases of the urinary organs in females and the urinary and sex organs in males.

V, W

Vasectomy: An operation to cut or tie off the two tubes that carry sperm out of the testicles.

Watchful waiting: Closely monitoring a patient's condition but withholding treatment until symptoms appear or change.

Appendix VIII:

Off the Bookshelf

Off the Bookshelf

Adam's Burden: An Explorer's Personal Odyssey Through Prostate Cancer, Charles Neider

American College of Physicians Home Medical Guide: Prostate Problems, Tony Smith

A Patient's Guide to Male Sexual Function, Tom F. Lue, MD

Dr. Patrick Walsh's Guide to Surviving Prostate Cancer, Patrick Walsh, MD, Janet Farrar Worthington

Hit Below the Belt: Facing Up to Prostate Cancer, F. Ralph Berberich, MD

How to Fight Prostate Cancer & Win, William Fischer

Humanizing Prostate Cancer: A Physician-Patient Perspective, Roger Schultz, Alex Oliver

Intelligent Patient Guide to Prostate Cancer, S. Larry Goldenbers

Mayo Clinic on Prostate Health, David Barrett (Editor)

Men, Women, and Prostate Cancer: A Medical and Psychological Guide for Women and the Men They Love, Barbara Rubin Wainrib

My Prostate and Me: Dealing with Prostate Cancer, William Martin

Natural Medicine for Prostate Problems, Ron Falcone

Oh No, Not Me! Prostate Cancer – One Man's Experience Told in Layman's Terms, Joseph Lintzenich

Prostate & Cancer: A Family Guide to Diagnosis, Treatment & Survival, Sheldon Marks, MD, Judd Moul

Prostate Cancer: A Non-Surgical Perspective, Kent Wallner

Prostate Cancer: New Medical Therapies, Lisa Henderson

Prostate Cancer: Overcoming Denial with Action, Allen Salowe

Prostate Cancer: Treatment Guidelines for Patients, American Cancer Society and National Comprehensive Cancer Network

Prostate Cancer Treatment Options: A Guide to the Basics, Will Connell

Prostate Cancer: What I Found Out & What You Should Know, Robert Maddox, Robert Dole

Prostate Cancer: What Every Man—And His Family—Need to Know, David Bostwick

Prostate Health in 90 Days: Cure Your Prostate Now Without Drugs or Surgery, Larry Clapp, PhD

Prostate: Questions and Answers You Have ... Answers You Need, Sandra Salmans

Protecting the Prostate, Karolyn Gazella

The ABCs of Advanced Prostate Cancer, Mark Moyad, Kenneth Pienta

The ABCs of Nutrition & Supplements for Prostate Cancer, Mark Moyad

Off the Bookshelf

The ABCs of Prostate Cancer: The Book That Could Save Your Life, Joesph Oesterling

The American Cancer Society: Prostate Cancer, David Bostwick

The Best Options for Diagnosing and Treating Prostate Cancer, James Lewis, Jr., PhD

The Healthy Prostate: A Doctor's Comprehensive Program for Preventing and Treating Common Prostate Problems, Arnold Fox, Barry Fox

The Herbal Remedy for Prostate Cancer, James Lewis, Jr.

The Lovin' Ain't Over: The Couple's Guide to Better Sex After Prostate Disease, Ralph and Barbara Alterowitz

The Men's Club: How to Lose Your Prostate Without Losing Your Sense of Humor, Bert Gottlieb, Thomas Mawn

The Natural Prostate Cure, Roger Mason

The Patient's Guide to Prostate Cancer: An Expert's Successful Treatment Strategies and Options, Marc Garnick

The Prostate: A Guide for Men and the Women Who Love Them, Patrick Walsh, MD, Janet Farrar Worthington

The Prostate Cancer Answer Book: An Unbiased Guide to Treatment Choices, Marion Morra

The Prostate Cancer Protection Plan: The Foods, Supplements, and Drugs that Can Combat Prostate Cancer, Bob Arnot, MD

The Prostate Cancer Sourcebook: How to Make Informed Treatment Choices, Marcus Loo, Marian Betancourt

"I Flunked My PSA!"

The Prostate Diet Cookbook: Cancer-Fighting Foods for a Healthy Prostate, Buffy Sanders, Michael Brawer

The Prostate: Everything You Need to Know, Adrian Wallwe, PhD

The Prostate Miracle: New Natural Therapies That Can Save Your Life, Jesse Stoff, PhD

Seeds of Hope: A Physician's Personal Triumph over Prostate Cancer, Michael Dorso

What Can I Do? My Husband Has Prostate Cancer, Bev Farmer

You Can't Make Love If You're Dead: Curing Prostate Cancer and Keeping My Sexuality, Leon Prochnik

Off the Bookshelf

My Notes

"Resources That Have Helped Me"
(And that I should recommend to others!)

_____
_____
_____
_____
_____
_____
_____
_____
_____
_____
_____
_____
_____
_____

Appendix IX:

Internet Resources

Internet Resources

The following Internet resources are not all-inclusive. Also, given the progressive nature of the Internet, a web site's address, content, or even existence may change. We suggest that you use this listing as a starting point for developing your own personal Internet resource list.

Ablin Foundation for Cancer Research
www.prostatefoundation.org

Affirming the Darkness: Prostate Cancer
www.affirming.com

American Cancer Society
www.cancer.org

American Prostate Society
www.ameripros.org

As We See It
www.prostatestories.com

California Prostate Cancer Coalition
www.prostatecalif.com

CaP CURE
www.capcure.org

Center for Holistic Urology
www.holisticurology.com

Iranian Prostate Cancer Society
www.iranianprostatesociety.com

Johns Hopkins Prostate Bulletin
www.hopkinsprostate.com

Malecare
www.malecare.org

Male Health Center, The
www.malehealthcenter.com

My Prostate and Me: Dealing with Prostate Cancer
www.ruf.rice.edu/~wcm

National Cancer Institute
www.nci.nih.gov

National Prostate Cancer Coalition
www.4npcc.org

PROstart Initiative
www.prostartonline.com

Prostate Cancer
www.mdanderson.org/diseases/prostate

Prostate Cancer: A Journey of Hope
www.pbs.org/ketc/prostatecancer

Prostate Cancer: A Survivor's Guide
pcaguide.com

Prostate Cancer Genetic Research Study (PROGRESS)
www.fhcrc.org/science/phs/progress_study

Prostate Cancer InfoLink
www.phoenix5.org/Infolink/index.html

Prostate Cancer News on the Net
www.cancernews.com/male.htm

Prostate Cancer Research Institute
www.prostate-cancer.org

Internet Resources

Prostate Cancer Research Network
pcrn.org

Prostate Cancer Risk Assessment Program
www.fccc.edu/clinicalresearch/prostateriskassessment/prostate.html

Prostate Health Directory, The
www.prostatehealthdirectory.com

Prostate Health Resources
www.prostate90.com

Prostatematters.com
www.prostatematters.com

Prostate Pointers
www.prostatepointers.org

PSA Rising Prostate Cancer Magazine
www.psa-rising.com

Seed Pods
www.prostatepointers.org/seedpods

Society for Basic Urologic Research
godot.urol.uic.edu/~sbur

Urology
www.urology.med.umich.edu

US TOO International, Inc.
www.ustoo.com

Your Prostate.net
www.yourprostate.net

Appendix X:

National Organizations

National Organizations

American Cancer Society
1-800-ACS-2345

American Medical Association
312-464-5000

American Foundation for Urologic Disease
1-800-828-7866

American Prostate Society
410-859-3735

American Urological Association
410-727-1100

California Prostate Cancer Coalition
510-271-7997

Cancer Connection
626-359-8111

CaP Cure
1-800-757-2873

Consumer Nutrition Hotline
1-800-366-1655

Foundation for Hospice and Home Care
202-547-7424

Hospice Education Institute
1-800-331-1620

Kaiser Permanente Prostate Cancer Education Seminars and Support
909-427-6340

Man to Man
1-800-227-2345

National Association for Continence
1-800-252-3337

National Cancer Institute
1-800-4CANCER

National Coalition for Cancer Survivorship
877-622-7937

The National Prostate Cancer Coalition
202-463-9455

Prostate Cancer Information
1-800-543-9632

The Prostate Cancer Resource Network
1-800-828-7866

Women's Suffrage for Prostate Cancer Awareness and Support
1-888-776-2262

My Notes

"Other Helpful Organizations"
(Including local groups and programs!)

Index

Index

A

Acupuncture 71
Adrenal glands 7, 61, 133
Advanced disease 84
African-American men 9, 15, 17, 31
Age 8, 14, 31, 38, 63
Age-adjusted PSA 34
Alternative therapies 48, 68
Aminoglutethimide 133
Analgesics 71
Androgen 7, 17, 133
Angiogenesis 64
Angiogenesis inhibitors 64
Antiandrogens 61, 62, 133
Antibodies 27
Appetite 77
Aromatherapy 68
Asian diets 22
Asian-American men 31

B

Benign 8, 133
Benign (non-cancerous) prostate conditions 38
Benign prostatic hyperplasia (BPH) 18, 21, 23, 38, 133
Bicalutamide (Casodex®) 61, 109, 134
Bilateral orchiectomy 126, 127
Biofeedback 68
Biological therapy 64, 134
Biopsy 33, 134
Bladder 5, 134
Blood transfusion 56

Bone scans 65
BPH (See benign prostatic hyperplasia)
Brachytherapy 57, 58, 124, 127, 134
Brachytherapy seeds (approved) 60
BRCA1 16
BRCA2 16

C

Cancer 134
Cancer Information Service 25, 36, 70
Cancer vaccines 21, 27
Career 80
Catheter 134
Caverject® 128
Changing jobs 81, 111
Chemotherapy 64, 111, 135
Children 49
Clinical trials 69, 135
Codeine 71
Common prostate cancer drugs 107, 111
Common anti-nausea medications 115
Communication 124
Complementary and alternative therapies 65, 68, 71
Complete androgen blockade 61, 126, 135
Computerized tomography (CT) 65
Cryoablation 64
Cryosurgery 64, 135
Cystoscopy 135

D

Depression 78, 121, 122
Dexamethasone 116
Diagnosis 43
Diet 16, 22
Dietary habits 13
Dietary supplements 25, 48
Digital rectal exam (DRE) 14, 31, 33, 135
Dihydroxytestosterone (DHT) 23
Docetaxel (Taxotere®) 112

Index

Dolasetron (Anzemet®) 116
Dry orgasm 57, 135

E

Early detection 31
Ejaculation 135
Emotional issues 78
Epoitin alfa (Procrit®) 112
Erectile dysfunction 79, 128
Estramustine phosphate (EMCYT®) 112
Etoposide (VePesid®) 112
Exercise 21, 77
Exhaustion 78
External beam radiation therapy 57, 58, 123, 127, 136
Externally assisted devices 128

F

False positive/false negative results 33
Family and friends 46
Family history 14, 15, 31
Fat 26
Fatigue 78
Fear of recurrence 77
Fentanyl patch 71
Financial issues 79
Finasteride (Proscar®) 21, 23, 136
Flare 62
Flaxseed 68
Flutamide (Eulexin®) 61, 109, 136
Free PSA 34

G

Garlic 25
Genes 15, 136
Gene therapy 63
Genetic risk 15
Genitourinary system 136
Gleason score 46, 100, 101, 102, 103
Goserelin (Zolodex®) 61, 108, 136
Grade 136

Granisetron (Kytril®) 116
Guided imagery 68

H

Herbal supplements 49, 71
Herbs 48
Hereditary factors 8, 15
High risk 102
High-fat diet 9
Hispanics 36
Hormonal agents 107
Hormonal therapy 61, 136
Hormones 7, 17, 137
Hot flashes 62
Hybritech® 34
Hydrocodone 71
Hydromorphone 71

I

Implant radiation 57, 58, 124, 127, 134
Impotence 57, 58, 62, 137
Incontinence 137
Intermediate risk 101
Implant or internal radiation 57, 137
Intimacy 78
Intravenous pyelogram 137
Isoflavones 26

K

Ketoconazole (Nizoral®) 61, 109, 137

L

Lack of exercise 9
Laparoscopic radical prostatectomy 56
Leuprolide (Lupron®) 61, 108, 137
Levorphanol 71
LH-RH agonists 61, 62, 138
Lifestyle factors 21
Local therapy 57, 137
Low risk 100

Index

Luteinizing hormone-releasing hormone (LH-RH) agonists 61, 62, 138
Lycopene 26
Lymph node 138
Lymphatic system 8, 138

M

Magnetic resonance imaging (MRI) 65
Malignant 8, 138
Massage 68
Medical oncologist 138
Megadoses of vitamins or minerals 48, 68
Megestrol acetate (Megace®) 109
Meperidine 71
Metastasis 7, 138
Methadone 71
Metoclopramide 116
Minority screening 36
Mitoxantrone (Novantrone®) 113
Morphine 71

N

Nerve sparing prostatectomy 55
Nilutamide (Nilandron®) 109
Nonprescription pain relievers 71
Nutrition 68, 77

O

Ondansetron (Zofran®) 116
Opioid narcotics 71
Orchiectomy 61, 62, 126

P

Pain 71
Paclitaxel (Taxol®) 113
PAP 33
Pathologist 139
PC-SPES 68
Pelvic lymph node dissection 55
Perineal prostatectomy 55
Personal support 82

Physical side effects 125
Prescription pain relievers 71
Prevention 21
Prochlorperazine (Compazine®) 117
Prostate Cancer Outcomes Study 54, 64
Prostate Cancer Prevention Trial 21, 23
Prostate gland 5, 139
Prostate, Lung, Colorectal, and Ovarian Cancer Trial 39
Prostate-specific antigen (PSA) 14, 31, 32, 33, 139
Prostatectomy 139
Prostatic acid phosphatase (PAP) 33, 139
Prostatic intraepithelial neoplasia (PIN) 38
Prostatitis 38, 44
PSA (See prostate-specific antigen)
PSA density 34
PSA velocity 34
Psychological factors 121

R

Race 9, 15, 31
Radiation oncologist 139
Radiation therapy 57, 139
Radical prostatectomy 55, 56, 125
Radioactive seed implants (See brachytherapy)
Radiotherapy 57
Recovery 77
Rectum 5, 139
Recurrence 13, 84, 140
Relaxation techniques 71
Retropubic prostatectomy 55
Risk factors 13, 18, 21, 140
Risk reduction 28

S

Saw palmetto 68
Scrotum 140
Second opinions 50
SELECT Trial 21, 24
Selenium 24, 26, 68
Selenium and Vitamin E Cancer Prevention Trial 21, 24
Semen 5, 140

Index

Seminal fluid 5, 140
Sexual activity 79
Sexual desire 62, 121
Sexual dysfunction 121
Sexuality 78, 119, 122
Sexually transmitted viruses 9
Shark cartilage 68
Side effects
- of hormonal therapy 62
- of surgery 56
- of watchful waiting 54
Sildenfil (Viagra®) 128
Simulation 58
Smoking 9
Sonogram 32, 140
Soy 25, 68
Sperm 5
St. John's wort 27
Stages of prostate cancer 45, 89
Staging 140
Support 82, 83
Surgery 55, 128
Surgical implants 129
Symptoms 44
Systemic therapy 140

T

Talking to your kids 50
Testicles 7, 61, 140
Testosterone 7, 61, 127, 141
Transrectal ultrasonography 32, 33
Transurethral resection of the prostate (TURP) 55, 141
Treatment follow-up 72
Treatment options 97
Tumor 141

U

Ultrasonography 141
Urethra 5, 141
Urgency 57
Urinary catheter 56

Urinary incontinence 57
Urologist 141

V

Vacuum-assisted devices 129
Vasectomy 18, 141
Vasodilator therapy 128
Very high risk 103
Vinblastine (Velban®) 113
Visualization/guided imagery 71
Vitamin D 26
Vitamin E 24, 26, 27, 68
Vitamins and minerals 25, 68

W

Watchful waiting 7, 53, 54, 99, 141

Y

Yoga 68
Yohimbine 128